DEMENTIA AND PLACE

Practices, Experiences and Connections

Edited by
Richard Ward, Andrew Clark and Lyn Phillipson

P

First published in Great Britain in 2021 by

Policy Press, an imprint of
Bristol University Press
University of Bristol
1-9 Old Park Hill
Bristol
BS2 8BB
UK
t: +44 (0)117 954 5940
e: bup-info@bristol.ac.uk

Details of international sales and distribution partners are available at:
policy.bristoluniversitypress.co.uk

Cover design by Clifford Hayes
Front cover image: Edward McLaughlan MBE

To Agnes, Alice, Dennis, Edward, Joy and Wendy for showing the rest of us how it's done and to all the people living with dementia, their care partners and supporters, who made this book possible.

Contents

List of figures and tables

Notes on contributors

Jill Batty was born in the north of England and has spent most of her life in London, UK. She had a long career as a personal assistant and latterly as a massage practitioner. She married her husband Dominic in 1975. Jill is a full-time carer for Dominic, who has lived with Alzheimer's disease for 17 years and maintains a keen interest in theatre and the history of London.

Chris Brennan-Horley is Lecturer in Human Geography and former Australian Research Council DECRA Fellow at the University of Wollongong, Australia. The common thread running through his research is deploying qualitative GIS as a lively technique for transformative ends. He regularly contributes his mapping expertise to interdisciplinary research teams.

Anna Brorsson is Assistant Professor in the Department of Neurobiology, Care Sciences and Society, Division of Occupational Therapy, Karolinska Institutet, Sweden. She is primarily a qualitative researcher. The purpose of her research is to provide new knowledge of the conditions for participation in activities and places in public space and society outside the home for people with cognitive impairments/ dementia, and to identify possible avenues to increase accessibility and provide relevant support.

Sarah Campbell is Lecturer in Integrated Health and Social Care at Manchester Metropolitan University, UK. She is a qualitative researcher and is interested in the everyday experiences of people living with dementia.

Habib Chaudhury is Professor in the Department of Gerontology, Simon Fraser University, Canada and has extensive research experience in the field of Environmental Gerontology. He conducts research and consulting work in the following areas: physical environment in long-term care facilities, personhood in dementia, community planning and urban design for active ageing, and dementia-friendly communities.

Andrew Clark is Professor in the School of Health and Society at the University of Salford, UK. Much of his work focuses on ways of investigating neighbourhoods and place-based communities using participative and participatory methods.

Joanne Connell is Senior Lecturer in Tourism Management, University of Exeter Business school, Exeter, UK. Her current research on developing dementia-friendly practices is funded by ESRC/Innovate UK as part of the UKRI Healthy Ageing Challenge research programme. She has worked extensively with organisation in the visitor economy such as Visit England and Historic Royal Palaces.

Dennis Frost was born in New South Wales, Australia and was diagnosed with frontotemporal dementia at age 59. In 2014 he became involved in the Dementia Friendly Kiama project and was elected chair of the Advisory Group. Since that time he has been active in raising community awareness around dementia and been an advocate for all people living with dementia.

Ingrid Hellström is Professor in Caring Sciences at Ersta Sköndal Bräcke University College, Stockholm, Sweden. She has a background in clinical gerontological nursing, especially in the care and support of people living with dementia and their families.

Lynda Henderson lives in Gerringong, New South Wales, Australia and is the partner and carer of a person with dementia. She is a founding member of the Dementia Friendly Kiama Advisory Group and an advocate for Dementia Australia. She has worked extensively in disability education and advocacy, and since the dementia diagnosis of her partner has directed this expertise towards dementia.

John Keady is Professor of Mental Health Nursing and Older People, a jointly funded position between the University of Manchester and Greater Manchester Mental Health NHS Foundation Trust, UK. He leads the Dementia and Ageing Research team at the University of Manchester and is Senior Fellow at the NIHR School for Social Care Research.

Agneta Kullberg is Senior Lecturer and has a PhD in Public Health Sciences at Linköping University, Sweden. She has a clinical background as a district nurse. Her research is focused on health promotion perspectives on neighbourhood and people living with dementia as in the example of the dementia-friendly community.

Eric Macnaughton is Research Manager of the Building Capacity Project in Vancouver, Canada. He has a PhD from the University of British Columbia Interdisciplinary Studies programme, with graduate training in community psychology and 25 years of experience doing community-based research, evaluation, and knowledge translation in the field of community mental health. Most recently he was involved in the *At Home/Chez Soi* project, an initiative exploring housing and supports for homeless people dealing with mental health and addiction issues.

Atiya Mahmood is Associate Professor in the Gerontology Department at Simon Fraser University (SFU), Canada. Her specialisation is in Environmental Gerontology and community-based participatory research. Her research focus is on ageing, persons with disability, mobility, social inclusion/exclusion, physical environment and health.

Kainde Manji has a background in social policy, with a particular interest in personalisation of social care. She currently manages About Dementia, Age Scotland's National Forum for Policy and Practice for People Living with Dementia, funded by Life Changes Trust.

Wendy Mitchell was diagnosed with young onset dementia in 2014 at the age of 58. As an advocate and campaigner for greater awareness and understanding of dementia she now travels widely throughout the UK. Wendy's autobiography *Somebody I Used to Know* is a *Sunday Times* best seller and has been adapted for broadcast on BBC Radio 4.

Elzana Odzakovic is Senior Lecturer in Caring Sciences in the Department of Nursing, Jönköping University, Sweden. She has a clinical background as a district nurse. Her main research interests are concerned with people living with dementia and their everyday life in the neighbourhood.

Stephen Page is Associate Dean (Research) and Professor of Business and Management, Hertfordshire Business School, University of Hertfordshire, UK. His current research on developing dementia-friendly practices is funded by ESRC/Innovate UK as part of the UKRI Healthy Ageing Challenge research programme.

Lyn Phillipson is Principal Research Fellow in the School of Health and Society, Faculty of Arts, Social Sciences and Humanities at the University of Wollongong, Australia. Her research focuses on the development and practice of inclusive methods to support the engagement of people with dementia. She uses these methods to conduct research in the areas of stigma, health services and dementia-friendly communities.

Alison Phinney is Professor at the University of British Columbia School of Nursing in Vancouver, Canada, and Co-Director of the Centre for Research on Personhood in Dementia. She is known internationally for her work on dementia, meaningful activity, and ageing. She conducts research in partnership with community leaders and people with lived experience with the aim of supporting personhood and social citizenship of older people, especially those living with dementia and their families.

Kirstein Rummery is Professor of Social Policy at the University of Stirling, UK, with research interests in gender, disability, ageing and comparative social policy. Her latest book, *What Works in Improving Gender Equality: International Best Practice in Childcare and Long-term Care Policy*, is available from Policy Press (https://policy.bristoluniversitypress. co.uk/what-works-in-improving-gender-equality).

Kishore Seetharaman is a PhD student at the Department of Gerontology at Simon Fraser University, Canada. His broad research interests lie at the intersection of architecture, urban design, and disability, and his current research focuses on the influence of the neighbourhood built environment on out-of-home mobility and social participation of people living with dementia.

Louisa Smith is Research Fellow at the Australian Health Services Research Institute, Faculty of Business and Law at the University of Wollongong, Australia. Her research focuses on people with disabilities and complex support needs, and the development of participatory methods that enable inclusion and social change. She uses these methods to explore issues around transition, gender and sexuality.

Richard Ward is Senior Lecturer in Dementia Studies at the University of Stirling, UK. He is a registered social worker with a research background in the field of ageing and dementia studies. His research covers social care practice, dementia and place, dementia-friendly communities and the lived experience of dementia.

Elaine Wiersma is Director of the Centre for Education and Research on Aging & Health and Associate Professor in the Department of Health Sciences at Lakehead University in Thunder Bay, Canada.

Her research aims to tell people's stories in ways that challenge stereotypes and misconceptions of older people, particularly persons with dementia. Advocacy, inclusion and rights form the fundamental values underlying her work. She and Alison Phinney are the academic co-leads on the Building Capacity Project.

Acknowledgements

The editors wish to thank Christeen Winford and Jennifer Souter for allowing us to use their image of Edward McLaughlan's artwork for the cover. Our gratitude also to the team at Policy Press, who supported us, and showed great patience, as we developed the book.

The authors of Chapters 2, 5 and 7 would like to thank all participants who generously gave their time to the research. The work reported was funded jointly by the Economic and Social Research Council (ESRC) and the National Institute for Health Research (NIHR). The ESRC is part of UK Research and Innovation. The views expressed are those of the authors and not necessarily those of the ESRC or the NIHR. This work formed part of the ESRC/NIHR Neighbourhoods and Dementia mixed methods study (https://sites.manchester.ac.uk/neighbourhoods-and-dementia/) and is taken from Work Programme 4.

Introduction: Placing dementia

Lyn Phillipson, Andrew Clark and Richard Ward

Is there some*where* that dementia belongs? If we had asked this question 20 years ago doubtless the weight of responses would have emphasised institutionalised settings: hospitals, clinics and care homes. Such places would likely be secured, perhaps bounded by fences – places of containment and segregation (Steele et al, 2019), of care, but also control (Ward et al, 2008; Kelly and Innes, 2013). They may even be places where the occupants desired to be elsewhere, congregating at the doors or at the edges of the building (Chalfont, 2008), perhaps even making a bid to escape (Chatterji, 1998; Bartlett, 2007). It is far less likely those responses would have foregrounded outdoor or public spaces. Indeed, commentators writing at the turn of the new century were keen to highlight that public spaces were rarely considered appropriate for people with dementia (Blackman et al, 2003). On the whole, biomedically informed research on dementia considered independent movement beyond the home to be fraught with risk, often focusing on the prevalence and frequency of people with dementia becoming lost, but without considering what role the environment itself might have played in these situations (for example, McShane et al, 1998). Silverstein and colleagues (2002) captured the caring but paternalistic and risk-averse mood of the time: 'If someone with dementia can walk, that person can wander and become lost. If someone with dementia is missing, that person is lost. And if someone with a dementia is lost, that person is at risk of harm' (p 7).

Fast-forward to the end of the first quarter of the 21st century and much has changed. Arguably, if we posed our question now a more diverse set of responses would ensue. Hopefully a more diverse range of people would feel entitled and enabled to offer their perspective, revealing that ways of engaging and eliciting the direct views of people living with dementia have in themselves evolved a great deal (for example Keady et al, 2017). Yet, arguably the legacy of efforts to 'place dementia' still inhabit approaches to the condition. Consider, for example, the everyday language of dementia care practice, talk of 'admission and discharge', of being 'allocated a bed', 'awarded a place in day care' or deemed 'eligible for respite'. This is the language of 'placing dementia', of people being put in place, that fails to acknowledge the autonomy of the person, where decisions are taken for or about a person rather than with or by them. It is language that reminds us of the politics of place in dementia care, and how place and space can serve to structure and compound inequalities and to disempower people living with dementia. Perhaps unsurprisingly then, the history of the relationship between dementia and place is one of unequal power relations, of how power is often spatialised, and how control over place is frequently an expression of power.

In this book, we aim to shift and expand the focus from 'placing dementia' to 'dementia emplaced'. That is, foregrounding the significance of the situations and conditions in which people live and manage life with dementia beyond care settings. The particular focus is on outdoor, public and shared spaces. Many of the contributions to this book also concentrate on one particular site or scale, that of the neighbourhood. This focus is grounded in a tradition of place-based research, which has used the neighbourhood lens to facilitate understandings of life (Sampson, 2012) – but has rarely been used to provide insights into life with dementia (Keady et al, 2012). In the book, we draw upon a range of perspectives to explore and demonstrate the significance of place and neighbourhoods to life with dementia, to dementia care practice and to evolving policy ambitions. As such, we believe this book will be relevant to a wide audience, including students, academics, practitioners and policy makers, and, we hope, to people living with dementia and care partners.

Place through the lens of dementia

The cornerstone of our argument developed during this book is that dementia and place are co-constitutive, both discursively and experientially. In other words, ways of understanding dementia have produced certain approaches or constructions of place that in turn have shaped the lived experience of dementia and of care. Yet, what unites a great deal of existing research and commentary in the field of dementia studies is an ongoing failure to question or problematise place in the context of this relationship. A review of the existing research into dementia in outdoor, public and shared spaces highlights the scant consideration that has been given to the meaning of 'place' or the act of 'placing dementia'.

Symptomology and epidemiology

Much biomedically informed research has viewed dementia through a lens of disabling symptoms, deficit and risk. This is evident in the study of how people with dementia move through spaces, focusing on the quantification of reductions in capacity; diminished walking speeds (Callisaya et al, 2017), reduced decision-making abilities (Dommes et al, 2015; Fang et al, 2018) and reduced mobility (for example Oswald et al, 2010; Shoval et al, 2011; Kaspar et al, 2015; Wettstein et al, 2015). It is also clearly seen in the myriad of papers which focus on disorientation in time and place. Content analysis of police reports (Bantry White and Montgomery, 2015) and newspaper articles (Rowe et al, 2011), as well as surveys and interviews (Bowen et al, 2011) have documented and catalogued the negative impact of these 'getting lost behaviours' of people with dementia. Dementia's problematic relationship with place is so taken for granted that it is used in diagnostic and forensic processes; antecedents and features surrounding incidents of 'going missing' are used in autopsy reports to determine the cause of death and getting lost away from home is used to inform early discovery and 'protection' for people living with dementia in community environments (Furumiya and Hashimoto, 2015).

While some might argue that such studies have been useful to reduce harm, this pathologising spatial lens has also had a tendency to problematise outdoor places and mobility for people with dementia (MacAndrew et al, 2018). As a result, it has been argued that people with dementia require tracking and monitoring for their safety to participate in places outdoors (McKinstry and Sheikh, 2013; Ly et al, 2015; Mangini and Wick, 2017) or, depending on the severity of their dementia, may even require institutionalisation and segregation, restricting their free access to spaces for their own safety (Steele et al, 2019).

Many biomedical interpretations argue that the risk of getting lost or injured in outdoor settings, usually as a pedestrian, is attributable to the nature and severity of the dementia. The environment is viewed as a neutral, static backdrop or container in which a person with dementia functions (or, in fact, doesn't). However, there is also a stream of biomedical and epidemiological research that highlights the active role that the environment can play in increasing the prevalence or incidence of cognitive decline and dementia. Cross-sectional and longitudinal data have been used to explore associations between environmental features and cognitive impairment, including: proximity to traffic noise, air pollution or power lines (Ranft et al, 2009; Weuve et al, 2012; Tonne et al, 2014; Clarke et al, 2015; Tzivian et al, 2016); land use mix (Wu et al, 2017); amount of green space/vegetation (Brown et al, 2018); the walkability of the neighbourhood (Clarke et al, 2015; Cerin et al, 2017) and other characteristics of the built environment (Wu et al, 2015). Alongside the built environment, social characteristics such as area deprivation, crime, social connections and support (Lee et al, 2011; Watts et al, 2015; Friedman et al, 2017) have been associated to some degree with cognitive decline. While still framed symptomatically, this body of work conceptualises the environment as also having potentially therapeutic elements for people with dementia.

Place and therapeutic design

Therapeutic design in dementia studies aims to mitigate risk and threat in environments by focusing on the properties and features that can support people with dementia. In fact, environmental design, along with other behavioural interventions, is now emerging as a core part of non-pharmacological treatments for people with dementia (Zeisel et al, 2016). Informed by a critique of the biomedical approach by proponents of person-centred care (Kitwood, 1993) the dementia design movement has helped to raise awareness of the potentially malignant impact of the built environment in exacerbating disability. To compensate for the impact of ageing and dementia on a person's cognition, physical and perception abilities, evidence-based dementia design principles have been applied to reduce stressors in the built environment (Fleming and Purandare, 2010; Keenan, 2014). Interventions based on these principles have been shown to reduce dementia symptoms, including wandering, agitation, aggressive behaviours, and psychotic symptoms (Zeisel et al, 2003) and, more recently, also point to the value of design to support competencies rather than just compensate for deficits.

Like other areas of dementia research, therapeutic design has mostly been studied and applied in formal care contexts (Marquardt et al, 2014), with principles operationalised and applied through the use of environmental audit tools and checklists at both the design stage and for retro-fitting of specialist dementia care settings (for example Fleming and Bennett, 2017). However, more recently, this therapeutic lens has also been applied to outdoor and public spaces, including the assessment of public and commercial buildings (Fleming et al, 2017), land use strategies (Biglieri, 2018) and in the foundational work on urban design conducted by Mitchell and Burton (2010), which examined how local neighbourhoods could be designed or adapted so that people with dementia could continue to use them and enhance quality of life.

Place and human rights

Research in architecture and design for dementia is evolving to focus on more diverse environments and how the design of spaces, together with behavioural and social programmes, can support independent living (Topo and Kotilainen, 2009; Charras et al, 2016; Alzheimer's Disease International, 2020). It is also seeking to understand how physical and social environments can come together with care interventions to support the human rights and aspirations of people living with dementia. People living with dementia have the right to freedom of movement and liberty and to be supported to maintain an activity space of regular activities within their neighbourhoods (World Health Organization, 2015; Steele et al, 2019; Houston et al, 2020). These rights are being demanded through dementia activism and a potential for alignment with the disability rights movement (Thomas and Milligan, 2018; Shakespeare et al, 2019) and is evident in some, but not all, expressions of the international Dementia Friendly Communities (DFC) movement (Alzheimer's Disease International, 2017).

Place as embodied and relational

Despite the potential benefits associated with environmental interventions, work which focuses exclusively on design and access rights has also been critiqued as artificially dichotomising the social and material, treating both dementia and place as an abstract set of disaggregated characteristics. This separation is also inconsistent with the perceptions of people with dementia themselves, who have more clearly articulated an integrated view of the people, places and networks that are needed to make their communities more dementia friendly (Crampton and Eley, 2013; Smith et al, 2016).

Research which has focused more on relational, experiential or subjective experiences of place is more limited and has, in the main, focused on interiors and personal objects in institutional spaces (for example Buse and Twigg, 2014, 2015) and to a lesser extent the home space (for example van Steenwinkel et al, 2012). That which has explored the relationships of people with dementia with outdoor places and spaces has frequently been associated with participatory methods, providing opportunities for people with dementia to exercise influence over the research, directing spatial relations through approaches such as walking interviews and photo and video documentation. From these studies, we are provided with an alternative view of dementia in place, with opportunities to witness and engage with the daily acts through which people with dementia express their agency and belonging within their neighbourhoods. Through the use of these methods, we encounter representations of people with dementia with capacities, who participate in the retail economy (Brorsson et al, 2013; Brorsson et al, 2018) and in meaningful leisure activities (Innes et al, 2016). We meet walkers and way finders rather than wanderers (Brittain et al, 2010; Brorsson et al, 2011; Brorsson et al, 2016; Kelson et al, 2017) as well as active users of public transport (Hauger et al, 2019). We witness outdoor places and spaces as central not peripheral to the well-being of people with dementia (Duggan et al, 2008; Lloyd and Stirling, 2015). Rather than places of threat, this new literature highlights neighbourhoods as places where social connection, inclusion and support are not fixed but experienced as relational, dynamic and fluid (Clarke and Bailey, 2016; Herron and Rosenberg, 2017; Odzakovic et al, 2018; Ward et al, 2018; Clark et al, 2020). As such, there are grounds to argue that neighbourhoods merit closer attention in a dementia context.

The what and why of neighbourhoods in a dementia context

Broader research on neighbourhoods shows that they are multi-dimensional: amalgamations of social and physical, real and imagined spaces that can hold greater or lesser importance for different people. As the recent pandemic has shown, they can be locations where people unite against *external causes* or *incoming threats*. Neighbourhoods are sites of political and economic production and socio-cultural aspiration, evident, for example, in the language of campaigns and localised attempts at empowerment (Blackshaw, 2010; Moulaert et al, 2010; Horak and Blokland, 2012) or renewal and regeneration (Duncan and Thomas, 2000). Imagined neighbourhoods may be conceptualised in the future, or the past, perhaps framed by romanticised notions of a sense of community that has subsequently been lost. Neighbourhoods are also the product of wider and deeper socio-economic structural inequalities, with the potential to determine life chances, opportunities for interaction and social engagement (Forrest and Kearns, 2001; van Ham et al, 2012).

Older and disabled people, children, women, those living in poverty and/or with chronic illness have long been identified as more likely to be impacted by structures operating at a neighbourhood level (Smith, 2009; Pagano, 2015; Lager et al, 2016; Talen, 2018). The drivers of such different and frequently unequal experiences are varied and intersectional. In the case of older people, these include care responsibilities, limited opportunity for mobility (financially or physically), and leading neighbourhood-situated lives rather than being oriented towards a workplace somewhere farther away. Here, social gerontology has started to highlight the differing experiences of ageing in place (Burns et al, 2012; Buffel et al, 2013; Versey et al, 2019) and reminds us that neighbourhoods can affect older people beneficially as well as detrimentally (Buffel et al, 2014; Buffel and Phillipson, 2019). Yet, despite recognition of certain key issues (Keady et al, 2012), dementia policy, particularly in respect to dementia-friendly communities, has largely overlooked neighbourhood locations in favour of other types and scale of place – notably cities, towns and, more recently, rural villages (Hebert and Scales, 2017; Turner and Canon, 2018). Where neighbourhoods do explicitly feature in dementia-friendly literature, it is largely with recourse to environmental design or locally organised provision of support (Crampton and Eley, 2013; Smith et al, 2016; Heward et al, 2017). But, what about the experiential realm? The everyday, subjective level of engagement with the many different facets of neighbourhood seems to have been overlooked in dementia studies.

As Smith (2009) summarises, the benefits of ageing in place can include independence and psychosocial well-being afforded by maintaining an intimate knowledge of the environment; an opportunity to remain in greater control of the environment, often while experiencing 'spatial restriction' (see also Rowles, 1978). While not extensive, environmental gerontology has explored how factors such as a sense of place, attachment, belonging and control might intersect with personal characteristics, physical and mental health, household composition, location, length of residence, and socio-demographic characteristics including ethnicity, gender and class in understanding experiences of ageing (Harper and Laws, 1995; Peace et al, 2006; Rowles and Bernard, 2013; Skinner et al, 2014). Yet, how such observations apply to or resonate with people living with dementia remains less clear. Of course, the benefits of ageing in place are neither uniform nor equal for any group or community. In this we must be mindful of the pitfall of some ageing research and avoid viewing dementia as a homogeneous experience. Rather, the field of dementia studies needs to embrace a more nuanced understanding of how living with dementia intersects with other attributes and characteristics in neighbourhood life.

It is unlikely that a unifying definition of what a neighbourhood is will be found in the following chapters. Most of the authors start from an assumption that neighbourhoods are socially constructed, and to that end, collectively offer a critique of the ways in which neighbourhoods might be more commonly approached in dementia studies. Taking neighbourhoods as social constructs means moving beyond treating them as fixed, with standardised properties and compositions, or demarcated and defined by cartographic boundaries (Clark et al, 2020). As such, the chapters that follow are not so much interested in the characteristics of neighbourhoods and their relative significance to people living with dementia as they are in the question of how to understand dementia when viewed through the lens of neighbourhood.

A neighbourhood-centred perspective: emerging plotlines for policy and practice

A growing body of research into the neighbourhood-based experiences of people living with dementia and their care partners points to significant levels of unmet need (van der Roest et al, 2009; Johnston et al, 2011; von Kutzleben et al, 2012; Black et al, 2019). This research tells us that it is less medical or clinical needs that remain unmet and instead the struggle to manage day-to-day challenges of finding company and opportunities for sociability, managing the home and finances, and engaging in meaningful activity (Miranda-Castillo et al, 2010; Crampton and Eley, 2013). Internationally, research tells a story of people who are at risk of becoming cut off from the places where they live and consequently segregated from the wider world, as a result of being inadequately supported. Until now, dementia policy and practice has focused too narrowly on the individual, failing to fully appreciate how a person's setting and situation can provide significant resources and meaning, with the potential to bolster agency and social engagement.

Taken collectively, the chapters in this book thus provide the foundation for a 'neighbourhood-centred' approach to dementia policy and practice. Our argument for a shift in focus comes at a time of rapid change to the geography and spatial organisation of dementia care. As policy seeks to usher people from institutionalised care towards ageing in place in their neighbourhoods, so the framing and approach to dementia care has to evolve. We need to move beyond ideas, language and relationships that originated within the walls of institutions and re-compose not only how we practise care and support, but also how we understand dementia. In this context, recognising individuals living with dementia as being part of a wider system and network of relations is vital to the planning and provision of services and support.

Recognising the social contribution of people with dementia

This book makes an important contribution to an emerging call to progress from an 'impairment-led' to a 'capacities-oriented' approach to dementia (Dröes et al, 2016; Vernooij-Dassen et al, 2018). Many of the chapters offered here demonstrate how people with dementia actively engage with the people and places where they live and in so doing have a significant influencing role upon the open-ended and unfolding nature of their neighbourhood. Yet, such a focus reminds us of the intensely political context in which any discussion of the agency and contribution of people with dementia takes place. In the UK, as in many affluent western nations, a programme of cuts to public spending under a policy of austerity has left a gap where help and support used to exist. In this context, an emerging drive for self-management (Mountain and Craig, 2012; Toms et al, 2015) and peer support (Keyes et al, 2016; Carter et al, 2020) has taken place against a backdrop of retrenchment of public services and efforts to shift responsibility for health and care onto communities, families and the individual. This policy narrative of self-responsibility has an atomising effect on users of health and social care, but a growing number of commentators are taking issue with the thinking behind it, instead having recourse to a relational ontology that underlines the interdependent, nested and networked nature of care and support (for example Tronto, 1993; Kittay, 1999; Barnes, 2012; Chapman et al, 2019). A neighbourhood-centred perspective adds to this debate by demonstrating the significance of place. Not only do people living with dementia belong to a web of relations and wider networks that are vital to managing life with the condition, but those relations are emplaced and shifting over time.

Introduction to the chapters

This book weaves together four main strands. One strand consists of first-hand accounts of neighbourhood and community written by people living with dementia (Wendy Mitchell and Dennis Frost) or a care partner (Jill Batty, and Lynda Henderson with support from Louisa Smith). Two of the accounts come from Australia, the others from the UK. All four detail the fluid and changing experience of living with dementia and facing significant milestones in relationships with people and places. Jill (Chapter 3) discusses the experience of moving house with her husband Dominic and the relationships and connections that sustained them both during the move. Wendy (Chapter 6), a campaigner and dementia advocate, reflects upon the advent of COVID-19 and the impact it has had on her day-to-day life. No longer able to travel widely, she describes her growing intimacy with the village where she lives and new-found friendships and connections with neighbours and other locals that have emerged during lockdown. Lynda (Chapter 9) writes from the perspective of a same-sex relationship, as carer for her partner Veda. She reflects on the changes and continuities from their time as activists in the LGBT community to now advocating for social change concerning dementia. The narrative from Dennis (Chapter 12) focuses far more on the sense of community that he rebuilt after the social isolation that went hand in hand with a diagnosis of dementia. Central to this has been the transformative experience of participation in a local dementia community development project in a small seaside town in south-east Australia.

Another strand to the book is a collection of three chapters that draw upon a five-year international study of the lived experience of neighbourhood for people with dementia and their care partners. The Neighbourhoods: Our People, Our Places study (N:OPOP) (2014–2019) incorporated field sites in Scotland, England and Sweden and used a longitudinal design to better understand neighbourhoods and dementia over time and place. It is to date one of the largest and most in-depth studies of the neighbourhood experiences of people with dementia and is part of a larger five-year programme of research on Dementia and Neighbourhoods (Keady, 2014). In Chapter 2, Andrew Clark and colleagues emphasise the interconnected, networked nature of neighbourhood revealed by the project. Neighbourhoods, they argue, are 'malleable and fluid phenomena that are produced through a changing constellation of experience, processes and interactions'. The argument developed here challenges assumptions about what makes a neighbourhood and in so doing recognises the sheer diversity of what neighbourhoods can be. Chapter 5 by Elzana Odzakovic and colleagues is the second contribution from the N:OPOP study. The focus here is on people with dementia who live alone, a growing demographic in many parts of Europe and North America. The chapter makes a rallying call for specific consideration to be given to people living on their own with dementia. The authors question an overwhelming framing of single householders as socially isolated, and often depicted as lonely, instead showing how much more could be done to enrich people's lives. A third chapter (Chapter 7) from the N:OPOP study comes from Richard Ward and colleagues and sets out an argument for a performative approach to understanding neighbourhoods. Focusing on the social practices of people with dementia, they build an argument for the benefits of attention to the 'doing of neighbourhood'. This chapter calls on readers to recognise the crucial role of people with dementia in leading social change, creating more inclusive neighbourhoods through their presence in public settings and social situations.

Another strand of this book focuses upon the practicalities of getting out and about in local surroundings and considers opportunities to facilitate and improve this experience for people with dementia. In Chapter 4 Anna Brorsson reviews a series of studies which deepen our understanding of some key challenges that people with dementia face in their neighbourhood. Writing from the perspective of her discipline as an occupational therapist, Brorsson shows how a focus on specific environmental challenges can help inform different solutions while foregrounding the agency and problem-solving capacities of people living with dementia. The chapter explores how people manage the ever-changing relationship with their neighbourhood through processes of adaptation and by finding creative solutions to the situations that present themselves. In Chapter 8 Kishore Seetharaman and colleagues helpfully review existing literature and evidence on dementia and mobility beyond the home and draw together a conceptual framework using models developed in the field of environmental gerontology. The chapter highlights that agency, belonging, autonomy and identity are intimately tied up with neighbourhood movement and engagement for people living with dementia. The authors offer a deeper and more nuanced understanding of out-of-home mobility and a clearer appreciation of the role that practitioners and the built environment can play in supporting people living with dementia.

A fourth strand concerns community development in a dementia context. In Chapter 10 Alison Phinney and colleagues map out preparations for a dual-sited project taking place in Canada. The field sites are separated by 3,000 kilometres and represent very different aspects of the geography and culture of Canadian life. The authors provide an outline of the Canadian context for work on dementia-inclusive development and reflect on a series of key considerations for setting up such an endeavour, highlighting the value of being clear about underpinning values and principles for the work ahead. By way of contrast, Chris Brennan-Horley and colleagues (Chapter 11) share reflections on a well-established community development project, one of the first of its kind in Australia. Focusing on collaborative map making, the authors describe drawing in local residents with experience of dementia to help build a dialogue about inclusive neighbourhoods. The chapter reflects on the mapping process and what it brings to the bigger challenge of community development that aims to position people with dementia at the heart of the work. Brennan-Horley and colleagues use the learning from the study to reflect upon the meaning of place and neighbourhood, showing how map making brings place into focus in particular ways, tapping into the situated knowledge of people living with dementia. For the final offering, Joanne Connell and Stephen Page (Chapter 13) argue that creating dementia-inclusive tourism and visitor destinations can support people with dementia to continue to travel and explore the world beyond their own neighbourhood. Reviewing a series of recent studies, the authors reflect on what they have learned about engaging a large-scale industry to promote change and the more specific learning about what people with dementia find useful and attractive when thinking about holidays or shorter excursions. The work of Connell and Page represents a significant step towards a very different approach to 'placing dementia' and, as with many of the chapters, helps to envisage a world where dementia exists 'without walls'.

References

Alzheimer's Disease International (2017) 'Dementia Friendly Communities. Global Developments. 2nd Edition', *Alzheimer's Disease International*, available from: https://www.alzint.org/u/dfc-developments.pdf [Accessed 9 January 2020].

Alzheimer's Disease International (2020) 'World Alzheimer Report 2020: Design, Dignity, Dementia: dementia-related design and the built environment. Volume 1', *Alzheimer's Disease International*, available from: https://www.alz.co.uk/u/WorldAlzheimerReport2020Vol1.pdf [Accessed 9 January 2020].

Bantry White, E. and Montgomery, P. (2015) 'Dementia, walking outdoors and getting lost: Incidence, risk factors and consequences from dementia-related police missing-person reports', *Aging and Mental Health*, 19: 224–30.

Barnes, M. (2012) *Care in Everyday Life: An Ethic of Care in Practice*, Bristol: Policy Press.

Bartlett, R. (2007) '"You can get in alright but you can't get out": Social exclusion and men with dementia in nursing homes: Insights from a single case study', *Quality in Ageing and Older Adults*, 8(2): 16–26.

Biglieri, S. (2018) 'Implementing dementia-friendly land use planning: An evaluation of current literature and financial implications for greenfield development in suburban Canada', *Planning Practice and Research*, 33(3): 264–90.

Black, B., Johnston, D., Leoutsakos, J., Reuland, M., Kelly, J., Amjad, H., Davis, K., Willink, A., Sloan, D., Lyketsos, C. and Samus, Q. (2019) 'Unmet needs in community-living persons with dementia are common, often non-medical and related to patient and caregiver characteristics', *International Psychogeriatrics*, 31(11): 1643–54.

Blackman, T., Mitchell, L., Burton, E., Jenks, M., Parsons, M., Raman, S. and Williams, K. (2003) 'The accessibility of public spaces for people with dementia: A new priority for the "open city"', *Disability and Society*, 18(3): 357–71.

Blackshaw, T. (2010) 'Community as place', in Blackshaw, T. (ed) *Key Concepts in Community Studies*, London: Sage, pp 83–9.

Bowen, M., Mckenzie, B., Steis, M. and Rowe, M. (2011) 'Prevalence of and antecedents to dementia-related missing incidents in the community', *Dementia and Geriatric Cognitive Disorders*, 31(6): 406–12.

Brittain, K., Corner, L., Robinson, L. and Bond, J. (2010) 'Ageing in place and technologies of place: The lived experience of people with dementia in changing social, physical and technological environments', in Joyce, K. and Loe, M. (eds) *Technogenarians: Studying Health and Illness Through an Ageing, Science, and Technology Lens*, Chichester: Wiley-Blackwell, pp 97–111.

Brorsson, A., Öhman, A., Cutchin, M. and Nygård, L. (2013) 'Managing critical incidents in grocery shopping by community-living people with Alzheimer's disease', *Scandinavian Journal of Occupational Therapy*, 20(4): 292–301.

Brorsson, A., Öhman, A., Lundberg, S., Cutchin, M.P. and Nygård, L. (2018) 'How accessible are grocery shops for people with dementia? A qualitative study using photo documentation and focus group interviews', *Dementia*, 10(4): 587–602.

Brorsson, A., Öhman, A., Lundberg, S. and Nygård, L. (2011) 'Accessibility in public space as perceived by people with Alzheimer's disease', *Dementia*, 10(4): 587–602.

Brorsson, A., Öhman, A., Lundberg, S. and Nygård, L. (2016) 'Being a pedestrian with dementia: A qualitative study using photo documentation and focus group interviews', *Dementia*, 15(5): 1124–40.

Brown, S.C., Perrino, T., Lombard, J., Wang, K., Toro, M., Rundek, T., Gutierrez, C.M., Dong, C., Plater-Zyberk, E., Nardi, M.I., Kardys, J. and Szapocznik, J. (2018) 'Health disparities in the relationship of neighborhood greenness to mental health outcomes in 249,405 U.S. medicare beneficiaries', *International Journal of Environmental Research and Public Health*, 15(3): 430.

Buffel, T., De Donder, L., Phillipson, C., De Witte, N., Dury, S. and Verté, D. (2014) 'Place attachment among older adults living in four communities in Flanders, Belgium', *Housing Studies*, 29(6): 800–22.

Buffel, T. and Phillipson, C. (2019) 'Ageing in a gentrifying neighbourhood: Experiences of community change in later life', *Sociology*, 53(6): 987–1004.

Buffel, T., Phillipson, C. and Scharf, T. (2013) 'Experiences of neighbourhood exclusion and inclusion among older people living in deprived inner-city areas in Belgium and England', *Ageing and Society*, 33(1): 89–109.

Burns, V.F., Lavoie, J.P. and Rose, D. (2012) 'Revisiting the role of neighbourhood change in social exclusion and inclusion of older people', *Journal of Aging Research*, 2012: 1–12.

Buse, C. and Twigg, J. (2014) 'Women with dementia and their handbags: Negotiating identity, privacy and "home" through material culture', *Journal of Aging Studies*, 30: 14–22.

Buse, C. and Twigg, J. (2015) 'Materialising memories: Exploring the stories of people with dementia through dress', *Ageing and Society*, 36(6): 1115–35.

Callisaya, M.L., Launay, C.P., Srikanth, V.K., Verghese, J., Allali, G. and Beauchet, O. (2017) 'Cognitive status, fast walking speed and walking speed reserve – the Gait and Alzheimer Interactions Tracking (GAIT) study', *GeroScience*, 39(2): 231–39.

Carter, G., Monaghan, C. and Santin, O. (2020) 'What is known from the existing literature about peer support interventions for carers of individuals living with dementia: A scoping review', *Health and Social Care in the Community*, 28(4): 1134–51.

Cerin, E., Rainey-Smith, S.R., Ames, D., Lautenschlager, N.T., Macaulay, S.L., Fowler, C., Robertson, J.S., Rowe, C.C., Maruff, P., Martins, R.N., Masters, C.L. and Ellis, K.A. (2017) 'Associations of neighborhood environment with brain imaging outcomes in the Australian Imaging, Biomarkers and Lifestyle cohort', *Alzheimer's and Dementia*, 13(4): 388–98.

Chalfont, G. (2008) 'The dementia care garden: Innovation in design and practice', *Journal of Dementia Care*, 16(1): 18–20.

Chapman, M., Philip, J. and Komesaroff, P. (2019) 'Towards an ecology of dementia: A manifesto', *Bioethical Inquiry*, 16: 209–16.

Charras, K., Eynard, C. and Viatour, G. (2016) 'Use of space and human rights: Planning dementia friendly settings', *Journal of Gerontological Social Work*, 59(3): 181–204.

Chatterji, R. (1998) 'An ethnography of dementia', *Culture, Medicine, and Psychiatry*, 22(3): 355–82.

Clark, A., Campbell, S., Keady, J., Kullberg, A., Manji, K., Rummery, K. and Ward, R. (2020) 'Neighbourhoods as relational places for people living with dementia', *Social Science and Medicine*, 252: 112927.

Clarke, C.L. and Bailey, C. (2016) 'Narrative citizenship, resilience and inclusion with dementia: On the inside or on the outside of physical and social places', *Dementia*, 15(3): 434–52.

Clarke, P.J., Weuve, J., Barnes, L., Evans, D.A. and Mendes De Leon, C.F. (2015) 'Cognitive decline and the neighborhood environment', *Annals of Epidemiology*, 25(11): 849–54.

Crampton, J. and Eley, R. (2013) 'Dementia-friendly communities: What the project "Creating a dementia-friendly York" can tell us', *Working with Older People*, 17(2): 49–57.

Dommes, A., Wu, Y.H., Aquino, J.P., Pitti-Ferrandi, H., Soleille, M., Martineau-Fleury, S., Samson, M. and Rigaud, A.S. (2015) 'Is mild dementia related to unsafe street-crossing decisions?', *Alzheimer Disease and Associated Disorders*, 29(4): 294–300.

Dröes, R.M., Chattat, R., Diaz, A., Gove, D., Graff, M., Murphy, K., Verbeek, H., Vernooij-Dassen, M., Clare, L., Johannessen, A., Roes, M., Verhey, F. and Charras, K. (2016) 'Social health and dementia: A European consensus on the operationalization of the concept and directions for research and practice', *Aging and Mental Health*, 21(1): 4–17.

Duggan, S., Blackman, T., Martyr, A. and Schaik, P.V. (2008) 'The impact of early dementia on outdoor life: "A shrinking world?"', *Dementia: The International Journal of Social Research and Practice*, 7(2): 191–204.

Duncan, P. and Thomas, S. (2000) *Neighbourhood Regeneration: Resourcing Community Involvement*, Bristol: Policy Press.

Fang, C.-W., Lin, C.-H., Liu, Y.-C. and Ou, Y.-K. (2018) 'Differences in road-crossing decisions between healthy older adults and patients with Alzheimer's disease', *Journal of Safety Research*, 66: 81–8.

Fleming, R. and Bennett, K. (2017) Environmental Assessment Tool (EAT) Handbook, *Dementia Training Australia*, available from: https://dta.com.au/resources/environmental-assessment-tool-eat-handbook/ [Accessed 9 January 2020].

Fleming, R., Bennett, K., Preece, T. and Phillipson, L. (2017) 'The development and testing of the dementia friendly communities environment assessment tool (DFC EAT)', *International Psychogeriatrics*, 29(2): 303–11.

Fleming, R. and Purandare, N. (2010) 'Long-term care for people with dementia: Environmental design guidelines', *International Psychogeriatrics*, 22(7): 1084–96.

Forrest, R. and Kearns, A. (2001) 'Social cohesion, social capital and the neighbourhood', *Urban Studies*, 38(12): 2125–43.

Friedman, E.M., Shih, R.A., Slaughter, M.E., Weden, M.M. and Cagney, K.A. (2017) 'Neighborhood age structure and cognitive function in a nationally-representative sample of older adults in the U.S.', *Social Science and Medicine*, 174: 149–58.

Furumiya, J. and Hashimoto, Y. (2015) 'A descriptive study of elderly patients with dementia who died wandering outdoors in Kochi Prefecture, Japan', *American Journal of Alzheimer's Disease and other Dementias*, 30(3): 307–12.

Harper, S. and Laws, G. (1995) 'Rethinking the geography of ageing', *Progress in Human Geography*, 19(2): 199–221.

Hauger, G., Berkowitsch, C., Wanjek, M., Schlembach, C., Rohsner, U., Duschek, B. and Dominko, C. (2019) Challenges in transportation system to support independent mobility of people with dementia. *IOP Conference Series: Materials Science and Engineering*.

Hebert, C.A. and Scales, K. (2017) 'Dementia friendly initiatives: A state of the science review', *Dementia*, 18(5): 1858–95

Herron, R.V. and Rosenberg, M.W. (2017) '"Not there yet": Examining community support from the perspective of people with dementia and their partners in care', *Social Science and Medicine*, 173: 81–7.

Heward, M., Innes, A., Cutler, C. and Hambidge, S. (2017) 'Dementia-friendly communities: Challenges and strategies for achieving stakeholder involvement', *Health and Social Care in the Community*, 25(3): 858–67.

Horak, M. and Blokland, T. (2012) 'Neighborhoods and civic practice', in John, P., Mossberger, K. and Clarke, S. (eds) *The Oxford Handbook of Urban Politics*, New York: Oxford University Press, pp 254–272.

Houston, A., Mitchell, W., Ryan, K., Hullah, N., Hitchmough, P., Dunne, T., Dunne, J., Edwards, B., Marshall, M., Christie, J. and Cunningham, C. (2020) 'Accessible design and dementia: A neglected space in the equality debate', *Dementia*, 19(1): 83–94.

Innes, A., Page, S.J. and Cutler, C. (2016) 'Barriers to leisure participation for people with dementia and their carers: An exploratory analysis of carers and people with dementia's experiences', *Dementia*, 15(6): 1643–65.

Johnston, D., Samus, Q.M., Morrison, A., Leoutsakos, J.S., Hicks, K., Handel, S., Rye, R., Robbins, B., Rabins, P.V., Lyketsos, C.G. and Black, B.S. (2011) 'Identification of community-residing individuals with dementia and their unmet needs for care', *International Journal of Geriatric Psychiatry*, 26(3): 292–8.

Kaspar, R., Oswald, F., Wahl, H.W., Voss, E. and Wettstein, M. (2015) 'Daily mood and out-of-home mobility in older adults: Does cognitive impairment matter?', *Journal of Applied Gerontology*, 34(1): 26–47.

Keady, J. (2014) 'Neighbourhoods and dementia', *Journal of Dementia Care*, 22: 16–17.

Keady, J., Campbell, S., Barnes, H., Ward, R., Li, X., Swarbrick, C., Burrow, S. and Elvish, R. (2012) 'Neighbourhoods and dementia in the health and social care context: A realist review of the literature and implications for UK policy development', *Reviews in Clinical Gerontology*, 22(2): 150–63.

Keady, J., Hydén, L.-C., Johnson, A. and Swarbrick, C. (2017) *Social Research Methods in Dementia Studies*, London: Routledge.

Keenan, H. (2014) 'People living with dementia and the built environment', *Australian Journal of Dementia Care*, available from: https://journalofdementiacare.com/people-living-with-dementia-and-the-built-environment/ [Accessed 9 January 2020].

Kelly, F. and Innes, A. (2013) 'Human rights, citizenship and dementia care nursing', *International Journal of Older People Nursing*, 8(1): 61–70.

Kelson, E., Phinney, A. and Lowry, G. (2017) 'Social citizenship, public art and dementia: Walking the urban waterfront with Paul's Club', *Cogent Arts and Humanities*, 4(1): 1354527.

Keyes, S.E., Clarke, C.L., Wilkinson, H., Alexjuk, J., Wilcockson, J., Robinson, L. and Cattan, M. (2016) ' "We're all thrown in the same boat ...": A qualitative analysis of peer support in dementia care', *Dementia* 15(4): 560–77.

Kitwood, T. (1993) 'Towards a theory of dementia care: The interpersonal process', *Ageing and Society*, 13(1): 51–67.

Kittay, E.F. (1999) *Love's labor: Essays on women, equality and dependency*, Oxon, Abingdon: Routledge.

Lager, D., Van Hoven, B. and Huigen, P.P.P. (2016) 'Rhythms, ageing and neighbourhoods', *Environment and Planning A: Economy and Space*, 48(8): 1565–80.

Lee, B.K., Glass, T.A., James, B.D., Bandeen-Roche, K. and Schwartz, B.S. (2011) 'Neighborhood psychosocial environment, apolipoprotein E genotype, and cognitive function in older adults', *Archives of General Psychiatry*, 68(3): 314–21.

Lloyd, B.T. and Stirling, C. (2015) 'The will to mobility: Life-space satisfaction and distress in people with dementia who live alone', *Ageing and Society*, 35(9): 1801–20.

Ly, N.T., Hurtienne, J., Tscharn, R., Aknine, S. and Serna, A. (2015) 'Towards intelligent and implicit assistance for people with dementia: Support for orientation and navigation', *ACM International Conference Proceeding Series*.

MacAndrew, M., Schnitker, L., Shepherd, N. and Beattie, E. (2018) 'People with dementia getting lost in Australia: Dementia related missing person reports in the media', *Australasian Journal on Ageing*, 37(3): E97–E103.

Mangini, L. and Wick, J.Y. (2017) 'Wandering: Unearthing new tracking devices', *Consultant Pharmacist*, 32(6): 324–35.

Marquardt, G., Bueter, K. and Motzek, T. (2014) 'Impact of the design of the built environment on people with dementia: An evidence-based review', *Health Environments Research and Design Journal*, 8(1): 127–57.

McKinstry, B. and Sheikh, A. (2013) 'The use of global positioning systems in promoting safer walking for people with dementia', *Journal of Telemedicine and Telecare*, 19(5): 288–92.

McShane, R., Gedling, K., Keene, J., Fairburn, C., Jacoby, R. and Hope, T. (1998) 'Getting lost in dementia: A longitudinal study of a behavioral symptom', *International Psychogeriatrics*, 10(3): 253–60.

Miranda-Castillo, C., Woods, B., Galboda, K., Oomman, S., Olojugba, C. and Orrell, M. (2010) 'Unmet needs, quality of life and support networks of people with dementia living at home', *Health and Quality of Life Outcomes*, 8(1): 132.

Mitchell, L. and Burton, E. (2010) 'Designing dementia-friendly neighbourhoods: Helping people with dementia to get out and about', *Journal of Integrated Care*, 18(6): 11–18.

Moulaert, F., Swyngedouw, E., Martinelli, F. and Gonzalez, S. (2010) *Can Neighbourhoods Save the City? Community Development and Social Innovation*, London: Routledge.

Mountain, G.A. and Craig, C.L. (2012) 'What should be in a self-management programme for people with early dementia?', *Aging and Mental Health*, 16(5): 576–83.

Odzakovic, E., Hellström, I., Ward, R. and Kullberg, A. (2018) '"Overjoyed that I can go outside": Using walking interviews to learn about the lived experience and meaning of neighbourhood for people living with dementia', *Dementia*, https://doi.org/10.1177/1471301218817453

Oswald, F., Wahl, H.W., Voss, E., Schilling, O., Freytag, T. and Auslander, G.K. (2010) 'The use of tracking technologies for the analysis of outdoor mobility in the face of dementia: First steps into a project and some illustrative findings from Germany', *Journal of Housing for the Elderly*, 24: 55–73.

Pagano, M. (2015) *The Return of the Neighbourhood as an Urban Strategy*, Champaign: University of Illinois Press.

Peace, S., Kellaher, L. and Holland, C. (2006) *Environment and Identity in Later Life*, Milton Keynes: Open University Press.

Ranft, U., Schikowski, T., Sugiri, D., Krutmann, J. and Kramer, U. (2009) 'Long-term exposure to traffic-related particulate matter impairs cognitive function in the elderly', *Environmental Research*, 109(8): 1004–11.

Rowe, M.A., Vandeveer, S.S., Greenblum, C.A., List, C.N., Fernandez, R.M., Mixson, N.E. and Ahn, H.C. (2011) 'Persons with dementia missing in the community: Is it wandering or something unique?', *BMC Geriatrics*, 11: 28.

Rowles, G. (1978) *Prisoners of Space? Exploring the Geographical Experience of Older People*, Boulder: Westview Press.

Rowles, G. and Bernard, M. (2013) *Environmental Gerontology: Making Meaningful Places in Old Age*, New York: Springer Publishing Company.

Sampson, R. (2012) *Great American City: Chicago and the Enduring Neighborhood Effect*, Chicago: University of Chicago Press.

Shakespeare, T., Zeilig, H. and Mittler, P. (2019) 'Rights in mind: Thinking differently about dementia and disability', *Dementia*, 18(3): 1075–88.

Shoval, N., Wahl, H.W., Auslander, G., Isaacson, M., Oswald, F., Edry, T., Landau, R. and Heinik, J. (2011) 'Use of the global positioning system to measure the out-of-home mobility of older adults with differing cognitive functioning', *Ageing and Society*, 31(5): 849–69.

Silverstein, N., Tobin, T. and Flaherty, G. (2002) *Dementia and Wandering Behavior: Concern for the Lost Elder*, New York: Springer.

Skinner, M.W., Cloutier, D. and Andrews, G.J. (2014) 'Geographies of ageing', *Progress in Human Geography*, 39(6): 776–99.

Smith, A.E. (2009) *Ageing in Urban Neighbourhoods*, Bristol: Bristol University Press.

Smith, K., Gee, S., Sharrock, T. and Croucher, M. (2016) 'Developing a dementia-friendly Christchurch: Perspectives of people with dementia', *Australasian Journal on Ageing*, 35(3): 188–92.

Steele, L., Swaffer, K., Phillipson, L. and Fleming, R. (2019) 'Questioning segregation of people living with dementia in Australia: An international human rights approach to care homes', *Laws*, 8(3): 1–26.

Talen, E. (2018) *Neighbourhood*, New York: Oxford University Press.

Thomas, C. and Milligan, C. (2018) 'Dementia, disability rights and disablism: Understanding the social position of people living with dementia', *Disability and Society*, 33(1): 115–31.

Toms, G.R., Quinn, C., Anderson, D.E. and Clare, L. (2015) 'Help yourself: Perspectives on self-management from people with dementia and their caregivers', *Qualitative Health Research*, 25(1): 87–98.

Tonne, C., Elbaz, A., Beevers, S. and Sigh-Manoux, A. (2014) 'Traffic-related air pollution in relation to cognitive function in older adults', *Epidemiology*, 25: 674–81.

Topo, P. and Kotilainen, H. (2009) 'Designing enabling environments for people with dementia, their family carers and formal carers', *Dementia, Design and Technology*, 24: 45–59.

Tronto, J.C. (1993) *Moral Boundaries: A Political Argument for an Ethic of Care*, Oxon: Routledge.

Turner, N. and Cannon, S. (2018) 'Aligning age-friendly and dementia-friendly communities in the UK', *Working with Older People*, 22(1): 9–19.

Tzivian, L., Dlugaj, M., Winkler, A., Weinmayr, G., Hennig, F., Fuks, K.B., Vossoughi, M., Schikowski, T., Weimar, C., Erbel, R., Jockel, K.H., Moebus, S., Hoffmann, B. and Heinz Nixdorf Recall Study Investigative, G. (2016) 'Long-term air pollution and traffic noise exposures and mild cognitive impairment in older adults: A cross-sectional analysis of the Heinz Nixdorf Recall Study', *Environmental Health Perspectives*, 124(9): 1361–8.

van der Roest, H., Meiland, F., Comijs, H., Derksen, E., Jansen, A., Van Hout, H., Jonker, C. and Dröes, R. (2009) 'What do community-dwelling people with dementia need? A survey of those who are known to care and welfare services', *International Psychogeriatrics*, 21(5): 949–65.

van Ham, M., Manley, D., Bailey, N., Simpson, L. and Maclennan, D. (2012) *Neighbourhood Effects Research: New Perspectives*, Dordrecht: Springer.

van Steenwinkel, I., Baumers, S. and Heylighen, A. (2012) 'Home in later life: A framework for the architecture of home environments', *Home Cultures*, 9(2): 219–20.

Vernooij-Dassen, M., Moniz-Cook, E. and Jeon, Y. (2018) 'Social health in dementia care: Harnessing an applied research agenda', *International Psychogeriatrics*, 30(6): 775–8.

Versey, H.S., Murad, S., Willems, P. and Sanni, M. (2019) 'Beyond housing: Perceptions of indirect displacement, displacement risk, and aging precarity as challenges to aging in place in gentrifying cities', *International Journal of Environmental Research and Public Health*, 16(23): 4633.

von Kutzleben, M., Schmid, W., Halck, M., Holle, B. and Bartholoeyczik, S. (2012) 'Community-dwelling persons with dementia: What do they need? What do they demand? What do they do? A systematic review on the subjective experiences of persons with dementia', *Aging and Mental Health*, 16(3): 378–90.

Ward, R., Clark, A., Campbell, S., Graham, B., Kullberg, A., Manji, K., Rummery, K. and Keady, J. (2018) 'The lived neighborhood: Understanding how people with dementia engage with their local environment', *International Psychogeriatrics*, 30(6): 867–80.

Ward, R., Vass, A.A., Aggarwal, N., Garfield, C. and Cybyk, B. (2008) 'A different story: Exploring patterns of communication in residential dementia care', *Ageing and Society*, 28(5): 629–51.

Watts, A., Ferdous, F., Moore, K.D. and Burns, J.M. (2015) 'Neighborhood integration and connectivity predict cognitive performance and decline', *Gerontology and Geriatric Medicine*, January–December 2015.

Wettstein, M., Wahl, H.W., Shoval, N., Oswald, F., Voss, E., Seidl, U., Frölich, L., Auslander, G., Heinik, J. and Landau, R. (2015) 'Out-of-home behavior and cognitive impairment in older adults: Findings of the SenTra project', *Journal of Applied Gerontology*, 34(1): 3–25.

Weuve, J., Puett, R.C., Schwartz, J., Yanosky, J.D., Laden, F. and Grodstein, F. (2012) 'Exposure to particulate air pollution and cognitive decline in older women', *Archives of Internal Medicine*, 172(3): 219–27.

World Health Organization (2015) 'Ensuring a human rights-based approach for people living with dementia: Thematic brief', *World Health Organization*, available from: https://www.who.int/mental_health/neurology/dementia/dementia_thematicbrief_human_rights.pdf [Accessed 9 January 2020].

Wu, Y.T., Prina, A.M., Jones, A.P., Barnes, L.E., Matthews, F.E. and Brayne, C. (2015) 'Community environment, cognitive impairment and dementia in later life: Results from the Cognitive Function and Ageing Study', *Age and Ageing*, 44(6): 1005–11.

Wu, Y.T., Prina, A.M., Jones, A., Matthews, F.E. and Brayne, C. (2017) 'The built environment and cognitive disorders: Results from the Cognitive Function and Ageing Study II', *American Journal of Preventive Medicine*, 53(1): 25–32.

Zeisel, J., Reisberg, B., Whitehouse, P., Woods, R. and Verheul, A. (2016) 'Ecopsychosocial interventions in cognitive decline and dementia', *American Journal of Alzheimer's Disease and Other Dementias*, 31(6): 502–7.

Zeisel, J., Silverstein, N.M., Hyde, J., Levkoff, S., Lawton, M.P. and Holmes, W. (2003) 'Environmental correlates to behavioral health outcomes in Alzheimer's special care units', *The Gerontologist*, 43(5): 697–711.

2

Understanding the meaning of neighbourhoods for people living with dementia: the value of a relational lens

Andrew Clark, Sarah Campbell, John Keady, Agneta Kullberg, Kainde Manji, Elzana Odzakovic, Kirstein Rummery and Richard Ward

Introduction

This chapter explores what neighbourhoods mean for people living with dementia. While the built environment, and the economic and political apparatus they comprise of such as shops, services and localised campaigning, are certainly important, our attention focuses on how people living with dementia understand neighbourhoods as sites of relationally constituted ordinary or everyday social connection, engagement and interaction. The chapter outlines the nature of associations individuals have with the wider social sphere of their immediate locale and considers how these ostensibly geographical proximate (or local) social connections might support people to live as well as they might with dementia. In doing so, it considers why it matters to understand the socio-spatial dimensions of neighbourhoods as relational and interconnected phenomena and considers the importance of thinking about neighbourhoods as more than environments in need of intervention or modification in order to support people living with dementia.

How are neighbourhoods understood in the dementia literature?

In a review published in 2012, Keady and colleagues noted that a surprisingly small amount of literature has focused specifically on the importance of neighbourhoods for people living with dementia. The review identified three domains of activity: outdoor spaces, the built environment, and everyday technologies. The first examines how the outdoor environment can be better designed and/or modified to support people living with dementia. This includes work on the design of streetscapes and road layouts to better support mobility, as well as ongoing work to enable easier access to a range of different environments such as green and recreational spaces. A second attends to navigation and mobility of environments, such as shopping centres, hospitals, museums and grocery stores. The third investigates the use of technologies, including virtual realities, to support access to, or better develop, environments beyond the home (Keady et al, 2012). Since then, a considerable body of work has continued to investigate these areas (Sturge et al, 2021) and continues to provide evidence of the need to better understand why and how people living with dementia interact with their immediate environments outside of the home. While more work has started to turn its attention to the social dynamics of neighbourhood life (for example Li et al, 2021; Sturge et al, 2021, pp 6–7), it remains tempting to reduce the associations between dementia and the outdoor environment to a set of required modifications in the guise of, for example, improved navigability, accessibility, layout and appearance. Such a framing arguably has echoes of early human-environment models in gerontology that supposed a dependent relationship between an individual's ability to access environments and his or her competency (for example Lawton and Nahemow, 1973; Lawton, 1983). The idea of the neighbourhood as an ecological unit or phenomenon for study, as well as a particular scale of activity, service provision and social organisation continues to hold sway in some areas of planning theory, where the 'manipulation of the local built environment and social interaction can positively influence urban space and foster community life' (Schubert, 2000, p 118). Indeed, environmental interventions aimed at better supporting individuals living with dementia can be seen in the promotion, and critique, of a range of 'dementia friendly community' initiatives that adapt the environment and enable people living with dementia to continue to go outdoors (Mitchell and Burton, 2006; Charras et al, 2016; Biglieri, 2018; Arup, 2019).

Of course, neighbourhoods are more than physical locations for the delivery and provision of residences, commerce or support for health and well-being. They are sites of lived experience, imbued with memories, and made up of the minutiae of daily exchanges and interactions between individuals and groups (Cattell et al, 2008; Smith, 2009; Wiles et al, 2009; Poortinga, 2012; Blokland, 2017).

Individuals living with dementia who can continue to participate in neighbourhood-based activities may experience a range of benefits associated with increases in physical activity, social connections and interactions, as well as better well-being (Bartlett and Brannelly, 2019; Clark et al, 2020; Li et al, 2021; and see Chapter 8 for more discussion). They, and their care partners and supporters, are also reported to benefit from being able to access safe and secure environments and opportunities to engage in social and leisure activities often as part of a 'dementia friendly communities' scheme (Herbert and Scales, 2017; WHO, 2017; ADI, 2018; Chapter 13).

However, and of considerable importance, those living with dementia may experience a reduction in the range, scope and scale of their interactions with the world outside their homes (Shoval et al, 2011; Wettstein et al, 2015). Of note here is Duggan et al's (2008) work reporting on the experiences of 22 people with early to moderate dementia and their carers about the use of the outdoor environment, which found that while people living with dementia valued the outdoor environment for providing access to exercise, fresh air, emotional well-being and informal encounters with neighbours and friends, they ventured outside less frequently. Carers, meanwhile, reported that the impact of dementia was to decrease the frequency of outdoor activity and to limit the areas visited to those that were the most familiar. The result is a somewhat paradoxical 'shrinking world' phenomenon whereby people with dementia (and often their carers) withdrew into ever-decreasing social and physical worlds despite recognising that maintaining external links was beneficial for health and well-being.

That neighbourhoods might become more restrictive for those affected by dementia points to a need to reconceptualise them as malleable and fluid phenomena that are produced through a changing constellation of experience, processes and interactions. Understanding neighbourhoods as processes, undergoing constant production rather than as a fixed reality, resonates with how they have been understood in other disciplines, including geography (for example Massey, 2005). Indeed, as we discuss later in this chapter, there has been some attempt to reconceptualise space through a relational lens in social gerontology (for example Andrews et al, 2013), which indicates an alternative way of framing how neighbourhoods might be understood for those affected by dementia, and which demands some reassessment of what neighbourhood are, where they are located, and how they might be understood and experienced. For while there is an established logic to understanding that neighbourhoods begin 'as we leave our front door ... in public health terms, the concept of a walkable zone of experience is important' (Blackman, 2006, p 33; Odzakovic et al, 2018), we argue in this chapter that this can potentially limit the scope of possibilities for understanding them as networked and relational entities.

This chapter thus makes two contributions to extend our stock of understanding of neighbourhoods and dementia. First, it provides an empirically driven assessment of the ways in which neighbourhood-based connections and interactions might matter in a dementia context. Second, and drawing on arguments about the relational nature of space, we consider the implications of conceptualising neighbourhoods as networked and relational processes rather than material forms. Viewed as such, neighbourhoods might be understood as always in progress, and emerging from interrelations and embedded practices rather than a priori forms (Massey, 2005). As a result, this chapter also acts as a precursor to the arguments made in Chapter 7 about the agentic capacity and capabilities of people living with dementia to engage in the social life of everyday places. In doing so, the chapter invariably runs the risk of setting up an awkward, and perhaps specious, duality between the social dynamics of neighbourhoods on the one hand, and their physical or material properties on the other, while also appearing to ignore the structural, historical, political and economic underpinnings that produce neighbourhood spaces and inevitably impact on how different groups experience them. Our intention is not to jettison alternative readings of what neighbourhoods might be, nor to ignore other dimensions of the lived experiences of neighbourhood life. Nor do we intend to descend into an overly romanticised, structurally naive view of what neighbourhoods used to be or what they could become. Rather, by foregrounding the relational, we seek to bring to the fore how a focus on the social, and explicitly *social production* of neighbourhood places, can provide opportunities for new ways of thinking about how neighbourhoods matter for people living with dementia.

Research design

The data presented in this chapter come from the ESRC/NIHR-funded Neighbourhoods: Our People, Our Places study. This investigated how people living with dementia and their families experience their lives at a local level (Ward et al 2018). It also explored the extent and nature of social and environmental interactions for those living with dementia and identified enabling and inhibiting factors for participating in the neighbourhood. The work was undertaken in three fieldsites in England, Scotland and Sweden. Participants were recruited mainly through third sector support groups in Scotland and England,

and through health and social care services in Sweden. Ethical approval was obtained for the research across all three settings via the applicable ethical governance systems in each locality, including the relevant NHS Health and Social Care panel in England. In keeping with the study protocol, all names reported in this chapter are pseudonyms.

Starting from a constructivist view of what constitutes a neighbourhood, participants were encouraged to reveal their own understandings and experiences of neighbourhoods through three methods. First, walking interviews in which people living with dementia and sometimes their care partners took us on a 'neighbourhood walk' and showed us around their local area. Here, discussion focused on memories of living there, as well as different connections to the place. Second, and considering home the starting point to a neighbourhood, we encouraged participants living with dementia to lead us on a filmed tour around their home (Pink, 2007). Finally, we used a participatory social network mapping technique to explore with family carers and people living with dementia (whenever possible) the relationships that they have in their 'everyday lives' and to consider with them how those relationships might offer opportunities for support, interaction and engagement (Campbell et al, 2019). The scope and scale of the data collected is detailed in Table 2.1, though it should be noted that the findings discussed here are drawn from analysis of the walking interview and network mapping data.

Findings

Adopting a relational lens to explore social phenomena recognises that individuals, experiences and things are 'continually being constituted and reconstituted through relationships' (Macdonald, 2019, p 205). So, in considering the relational properties of neighbourhoods for people living with dementia, we focus on two aspects (see also Chapters 3, 5 and 7). First, we examine the importance of relations that develop, often fleetingly, in local spaces outside of the home, which comprise of relations with neighbours, local acquaintances and *familiar strangers* categorised under the heading of 'support nearby'. Second, we consider how such relationships are themselves constituted through a relational sense of place that can facilitate belonging and inclusion.

Support nearby

Participants experienced their neighbourhoods as assemblages of connections to people, places and memories, as well as locations

Table 2.1: Participants' relationship/household structure and data collection by fieldsite

		England	Scotland	Sweden	Total
Participants	Total	54	47	26	127
	Living with dementia	29	22	16	67
	Nominated care partner	25	25	10	60
	Of whom …				
	Were living in a couple dyad	50	32	20	102
	Were living alone	4 (PwD)	6 (PwD) 9 (carer)	6	25
Age (of person living with dementia)	Youngest	57	51	62	
	Oldest	88	88	87	
Methods	Network maps	53	55	30	138
	Walking interviews	41	40	18	99
	Home tour	30	29	0	59
	Other	2 mobility diaries	5 mobility diaries 1 diary	0	8
	Total	126	130	48	304

Note: PwD = People with dementia

where they live, shop and access services. They described a diverse and complex range of different types and functions of local associations, including family, friends, acquaintances and familiar strangers that offer a form of connection, and subsequent support, through physical proximity and regular co-presence. Neighbours, for example, while described as people with whom participants were not overly familiar, could provide practical assistance and ongoing reassurance that ranged from the security of a *watchful eye* to practical input into relatively mundane chores. They undertook a variety of *utilitarian* acts, mostly associated with small or everyday favours such as managing household waste, taking in deliveries, tending to gardens, looking after pets and properties when residents were away, and keeping an eye out for anything untoward. Such activities make up what many participants described as good neighbourly practices:

Interviewer:	They're good neighbours.
Olivia:	What makes you say they're good neighbours?
Interviewer:	Because, the thing is, they bring my [rubbish] bin out [from the street] for me.
Olivia:	And do they do that without being asked, or do you have to ask them?
Interviewer:	No, no, they do it voluntary.

(Olivia, care partner England)

Susan:	We've got to know some of the neighbours, people on both sides are great, and the next door but one, and another lady down the road who works at our local supermarket; So ... they've made an effort to be friendly with us. Because when we were looking for a home we came to look at the house, and the lady next door invited us in for a cup of tea. And the day we moved in the lady on this side, they're a young couple ... brought a plant as a welcoming gift ... So the people on both sides are fantastic. We've always been very fortunate with neighbours ...
Interviewer:	So if you needed anything in an emergency do you feel that they are people you could call on?
Susan:	We could, I mean sadly the guy next door has got health problems as well, and it looks like he's now living with dementia as well as other physical health problems; and with [another neighbour] just having another baby we're reluctant to sort of bother them too much. But, yeah, I mean when we have to go away, on a business trip or whatever, [neighbour] looks after the dogs ... She's always willing to do that.

(Susan, living with dementia, England)

Interviewer:	Who looks after your garden while you're away?
Trevor:	M----- next door.
Sal:	It takes her hours to water all the pots and plants and ...
Trevor:	She's lovely though isn't she?
Sal:	I tend to like put all the pots and tubs and everything in one area and leave the hosepipe

there so she just has to ... then I put them all
back where they belong when we come home.

(Sal, living with dementia and care partner
Trevor, England)

These small favours maintain a degree of sociability and provide
'assistance that restricted to casual actions that entail few costs'
(Baumgartner, 1988, p 13) but they rely on maintaining a respectable
distance (Crow et al, 2002) or 'moral minimalism' (Baumgartner, 1988)
rather than an emotionally close connection. Few participants spoke
of developing intimate friendships with neighbours regardless of how
long they and their neighbours may have known each other. Rather,
neighbours occupy a simultaneously ambiguous yet normative position,
such that while there are seemingly implicit expectations about what it
means to 'know ones neighbours', or indeed of who or what constitutes
a 'good neighbour', it is not easy to articulate what these are:

Danny:	Well, I know the girl who lives next door because she grew up round here ... and we know a couple of them, but we don't know the surnames, do we?
Jean:	We know people to nod and that's it.
Danny:	But we don't actually know people by name

(Danny, care partner and Jean, living with
dementia, England)

Albert:	The couple next door, they're good ... They speak to you, but that's as far as it goes. That's all I want. I mean, I don't want anybody that's in your life all the time, you know, but it's nice to have good neighbours.

(Albert, living with dementia England)

Interviewer:	And have you got to know any of your neighbours here?
Adam:	Oh yeah.
Pam:	Either side we know reasonably well and we know probably most people who live along this road, but no. Obviously we're able to say hello and have a, kind of, just a general chat, you know, but it's not close friends.

(Adam, living with dementia, and Pam, care
partner England)

This recognition without intimate familiarity underpins good neighbourly practices and produces a somewhat taken-for-granted social order that can contribute to a sense of belonging in place that has been identified previously (Bulmer, 1986; Crow et al, 2002; van Eijk, 2012). Shallow or informal interactions with others who live, or even work, locally can range from the subtlety of a smile through a window or an acknowledgement of presence when passing by, through to clear recognition and a stop for a chat on the street or over a garden fence (Blokland, 2003). This does not make such weak ties any less significant than stronger ones, for in the case of those living with dementia, they can take on a particular symbolic quality through their implied, as well as realised, ongoing social connectivity.

Beyond this, connections to neighbours also bring a sense of security and of help being available should it be required, and on occasions when assistance is needed (such as when a participant living with dementia might leave the house unaccompanied and unannounced, or become disoriented when alone outdoors), then neighbours are often the first port of call. As Douglas explains, neighbours can thus provide a 'safety net' of support (Wiersma and Denton, 2016) that, while perhaps rarely used, is not redundant:

Douglas:	I don't really visit people you know. I just see them when they pass, they are just next door people. I just talk to them because they are my neighbours.
Interviewer:	And are they helpful neighbours to have?
Douglas:	Yeah, yeah, they are very friendly.
Interviewer:	And do they do anything to help you?
Douglas:	Well, you see I don't really ask them for help. You know ... I don't need to, you know ... But if I ever need to, I could always ask her, you know.

(Douglas, living with dementia, Scotland)

Neighbourly activities are not unilaterally 'done to' those living with dementia. Nor do they happen organically. Rather, maintaining good relations with neighbours requires emotional and social labour as well as reciprocated effort from all parties:

Judy:	And Beatrice lives down there on the right, so yeah.
Interviewer:	Are these all friends that you've made since ...
Judy:	Since coming up here, yes.
Interviewer:	So you're quite integrated in the community?

Judy:	Yes.
Frank:	But it's hard work.
Interviewer:	And it's something that you've worked at.
Frank:	Well, I don't think consciously, actually, but it's just fairly naturally sort of ... outward going people, I don't know. I learned a very long time ago that you can't expect people to be friendly to you if you're not friendly to them, so it's very much a two way [street].

(Judy, living with dementia and Frank, care partner, Scotland)

In sum, interactions between participants and their neighbours, and the relationships such interactions come to reproduce, are conducted at a polite distance. Neighbours do not interfere or 'get in the way' (and those that do run the risk of being admonished for being 'nosey'), but this does not mean that they do not constitute an important part of a wider network of connections for those living with dementia. And while dementia might change the function of these relationships, for instance with respect to the sort of support offered, it does not alter the form these relationships take. For what matters for those individuals in our study is their sense that they are a part of these networks, rather than how well integrated they might be within them. The importance of neighbourly relations thus lies less in knowing everybody in the street, than knowing some people who are close enough to be called upon for support if needed.

Connecting as belonging

Local social connections have the capacity to act as channels for information sharing and social interaction, but also exist as relational webs of support; metaphorical safety nets available in exceptional circumstances (Wiersma and Denton, 2016). As reported in the previous section, neighbours can be a key source of immediate support and, because of their geographical proximity, often at short notice. Such relations are important for more than their seemingly utilitarian or practical value. The potential to interact, even occasionally, with a neighbour, or be recognised by face if not by name by those who live around and about, enable participants to feel connected to a wider social realm outside of the home, and subsequently feel a sense of belonging in and to place (Wiles et al, 2009).

Such belonging is achieved not just by being in a familiar environment, but through the recognition by, and the anticipation of being able to engage with, others. For instance, Lennart reflected on how exercising his pet dog also fostered a sense of connection brought about through familiarity:

Lennart: Since I have [my dog], I have become so popular because it is [my dog] who attracts people. When children come 'B- (name of the dog)' they shout, and we always get noticed.
                (Lennart, living with dementia, Sweden)

As Lennart implies, being recognised in the street or local shops offers an important sense of belonging in place, when a moment of recognition through a passing hello, smile, nod of the head or even brief eye contact reflects a connection with, and belonging to, place. Such individuals may be encountered on a regular basis but personal details, such as names, where they live or other intimate details remain unknown. Lily goes to a shop almost daily, ostensibly to collect a newspaper for herself, and occasionally, a neighbour. Her visits mean that she is easily recognised by store staff who 'look out for her' and ask after her health. Such exchanges are short-lived but their legacy, at least for Lily, enables her to feel connected to a part of a broader network of individuals. Indeed, when Lily was too unwell to make her regular trip to the store an employee delivered the paper to her home. Yet the value of such fleeting interactions may go unrecognised until they no longer exist, as Albert and Vera indicated when reflecting on Albert's trips to a nearby newsagents or 'paper shop':

Interviewer: When you go to your paper shop, are those people that you know, not know well, but [know] to have a chat to or …?
Vera: Yeah, but they don't know [Albert's] got Alzheimer's, no they don't.
Albert: … And the paper shop which I used to go to at the top of the road …
Vera: Oh that was great. It's closed now, they knew him very well there.
Albert: They knew me and I knew them. I could stop and have a chat with them, you know.
                (Vera, care partner and Albert, living with dementia England)

The closure of local shops and services, and indeed moving away (see Chapter 3) could all impact on the scope and scale of local connections, and point to an alternative albeit related sense of a 'shrinking world' as outlined by Duggan et al (2008). So too can dementia contribute to a seemingly shrinking world for participants in our own study. For instance, some described experiencing anxiety or a loss of confidence around leaving the home independently because of symptoms of the condition, such as memory loss or disorientation, or finding physical mobility more difficult. Such concerns need to be recognised, not least because of their impact on the ability to maintain social connections.

Implicit in the examples here is the way in which people living with dementia engage in a relational sense of neighbourhood connectivity. While the neighbourhood provides some supportive social infrastructure, it is experienced through a familiarity built up through traversing familiar networked routes rather than knowing a neighbourhood as a cartographic plane (see also Chapter 11). It is this networked familiarity, whereby neighbourhoods consist of a series of growing and shrinking routes and more and less familiar nodes, rather than presented as complete, map-like knowledge, that makes up lived experience. Neighbourhoods mattered to participants so long as they were able to keep up a regular and routine presence within them, 'getting by and getting on'. It was the process of encountering others, recognising individuals in familiar places at routine times of the day or week, and just as importantly, finding themselves recognised by others in familiar places and routine times, that was important.

Maintaining routines in time and place contributes to a much more networked, and, we suggest, fluid sense of how neighbourhoods are experienced. For example, Emily's husband Dylan cycles a regular route alone, while Suzanne follows a regular jogging route, which means both can draw support and find some reassurance from their neighbourhoods, which enables them to maintain a sense of independence, at least for the time being: "At the minute [Dylan] doesn't get lost but very often he can't now tell me the route he's taken …No, but we've always lived in this area and he's always cycled and run in the same area, so he's still using the same routes … So they're very familiar to him" (Emily, care partner to Dylan, England).

> 'I [run] in the park, which is just down the road, and into
> the village and … Depending on how far or how long
> I want to run I'll [go there] … and so far I've not got lost

or anything. I'm dreading the time when I'll suddenly think, oh no, where am I, I don't really recognise this bit?' (Suzanne, living with dementia, England)

Returning to Lily, a fortnightly visit to her sister-in-law allows her to maintain a sense of independence (see also Ward et al, 2018) and points to a more enabling relational personal geography:

'[From] the bus stop on the other side [of the street] I can go all the way to the shopping centre if I want and my sister-in-law lives in between … I don't go anywhere else on the bus, but I can go to her house. … I can do that no problem … I've done it for so long it's like going to the corner, you know.' (Lily, living with dementia, England)

Here, Lily evokes a familiar language associated with neighbourhood life, of "going to the corner" that relies on a spatial imaginary of localness that has resonance in much neighbourhood work, but with a notable difference. And as Lily's experience implies, neighbourhoods are not necessarily bounded spaces, defined by the walkability from one's front door. Rather, the capacity for familiarity means that those places farther away from home might be considered just as 'local' as those geographically closer, such that Lily's neighbourhood becomes stretched across space.

What provides the reassurance for those participants who are able to maintain connections to their neighbourhoods is thus the ability to recognise, and themselves be recognised by, others and this recognition itself depends on being able to maintain a set of mundane routines in time and space. Being 'local' is a prominent part of the discourse on neighbourhoods, and the relations with geographically proximate neighbours discussed previously certainly matter. A sense of networked familiarity also matters; of being able to navigate and belong to spaces and times that, while maintaining the hallmarks of 'localness', are geographically more dispersed. To illustrate further, some participants who had migrated to the UK maintained cultural associations with where they were born. This included regular contact with relatives overseas and acquaintances who had also migrated to the UK as well as maintaining cultural links, for example through visits to hair salons, specialist food stores and attendance at community groups providing culturally relevant activities. Such activities were seldom located within the immediate geographies of participants' local neighbourhoods and required (notably with support) travel and planning to attend them and maintain the connections. Finally, participant Ruth offers a stark example of the networked nature of where she felt she belonged:

Ruth: Now, I think my [number of] virtual friends are getting bigger. Isn't that amazing?

Interviewer: Yeah, that's interesting, isn't it?

Ruth: So my virtual friends are getting bigger, and I'm getting more work to do from my home, in Zoom meetings. Like this morning, Canada and various things like that. So the virtual friends are almost taking over.

(Ruth, living with dementia, Scotland)

Ruth had become increasingly involved in dementia activism and had become a member of a number of campaigning groups to improve support for people living with the condition. While Ruth's particular circumstances might have given rise to a more networked set of connections, her experiences also indicate the importance of questioning the meaning of place in the context of fluid social proximities.

Neighbourhoods as relational places

Neighbourhoods are locations where people living with dementia interact with individuals beyond the family and participate in a wide network of connections. In this sense, discourses around the apparent demise of neighbourly relations are perhaps overplayed, or at least are more nuanced. Nonetheless, recognising that ostensibly local social relations can be stretched across space requires reflection on how we can understand where, and what, a neighbourhood is for those affected by dementia. Relationality has started to gain popularity in dementia studies, including in understanding care (Clarke et al, 2020), but also in the study of communication (Hydén, 2017) and arts-based practices (Kontos and Grigorovich, 2018). It provides a lens through which to understand the reciprocal nature of selfhood (Kontos et al, 2017) and, perhaps above all, rejects the idea of discrete units such as the individual or society as the starting point for analysis (Emirbayer, 1997). In line with Andrews et al (2013), we posit that so too can neighbourhood relations and indeed neighbourhoods (themselves, assemblages of locations, activities and institutions) be understood relationally. Central to understanding neighbourhoods relationally is an awareness of the interdependency of individuals with others, demonstrated most clearly in the ways in which participants in our study experience and maintain connections carved in space and time. That such familiarity can be far from 'local' in a cartographic sense hints at how neighbourhoods themselves might be constituted and experienced as relational and networked processes for individuals living with dementia. We agree with Andrews et al (2013) that there is value in exploring how neighbourhoods are constituted as relational entities that grow and contract in different interactional contexts in relation to other places and scales. The experiences we have outlined here do not, necessarily, transcend great distances, nor even operate at very many different scales, but in the case of dementia, we know that distance and scale are malleable (Duggan et al, 2008), such that, as Lily put it earlier, even "going to the corner" can evoke quite different meanings. The encounters and connections that participants in our study experience are embedded in a sense of localness enabled through regular and repeated connection to and engagement with places regardless of distance. We need to approach neighbourhoods as local places, not in terms (for instance) of physical locations identified at the scale of walkability, but rather as transcending geography in order to maintain ongoing routines, senses of familiarity and social interconnectivity across multiple sites.

Andrews et al (2013) offer a useful critique of how space and place have been approached in some aspects of gerontology, taking issue with the somewhat depoliticised approach to space as locations in which people and other things can be located, mapped, tracked and measured. In the case of dementia, this might include the mapping of diagnoses (Tampubolon et al, 2018), the tracking and subsequent mapping of the movement (or lack thereof) of people living with dementia, such as with the use of GPS technologies (Wigg et al, 2010), work to improve physical activity (Alidoust et al, 2018) or research on how to monitor mobility (Lin et al, 2014; Hammoud et al, 2018). This work certainly contributes a vital evidence base for the development of well-intentioned interventions, policy and practice, including the important task of redesigning neighbourhood environments and the services that are offered within them. But in such work, space (and in this we might include neighbourhoods) are too frequently, and arguably implicitly, conceptualised as 'containers' to be navigated, within which activities take place such as engagement with other people and services accessed. Yet if space is 'networked and performed articulations of social relations' that consists of 'bundles of interrelations ... forever coming into being' (Andrews et al, 2013, p 1348), then we need to understand neighbourhoods through a rather different lens. Attempts to theorise why neighbourhoods matter for people living with dementia must go beyond models of environmental adaptation or behaviour change, checklists of barriers to be removed. Neighbourhoods are more than places 'out there', to be mapped, traversed or discovered lying just beyond one's front door. They are also more than containers of potentially hazardous or risky features and activities in need of being made 'friendlier' through removal or modification before those living with dementia can be trusted to venture into them. Viewing neighbourhoods as such runs the risk of reducing those living with dementia to the status of a vulnerable population only able to 'consume' such sites once they have been made safe by others. Of course, this does not mean that neighbourhoods are risk free, experienced equally or accessible to all. Nor is it to imply that those living with dementia do not need support to engage with them. Rather, approaching neighbourhoods through a lens of relationality emphasises how they come into being as processes, undergoing constant social production rather than existing as passive sites requiring modification. It also requires understanding how people living with dementia themselves are active in their production as sites of social connection and interaction.

Conclusion

This chapter has taken a twofold approach to exploring the meaning of neighbourhoods for people living with dementia through a relational lens. First, it has considered relationships and informal interactions beyond the home. Second, it has begun to outline how neighbourhoods might be relational places, compressed and stretched over space rather than as cartographic planes demarcated by clear boundaries. There is certainly something of a tension at play here between recognising the importance of geographically proximate relations in and to place, while simultaneously questioning the nature of what constitutes a local place. As such, questions remain about the slipperiness of a term like 'local' when understanding the meaning of neighbourhoods, and caution is required when conflating terms like community and neighbourhood, for instance in the development of various 'dementia friendly' initiatives. Understanding neighbourhoods relationally means abandoning attempts to compare and contrast different neighbourhoods for degrees of 'friendliness' or assessing whether neighbourhoods are any more or less supportive now compared to the past. For some people living with dementia, some of the time, 'local' connections and 'local' places are not necessarily geographically proximate and can be found in a different part of a town, overseas or online. So, this chapter serves as a useful reminder (if one were needed) that neighbourhoods for those living with dementia can extend beyond conventional expectations of where neighbourhood experiences are located. It is important to ensure individuals can continue to transcend locally bounded places to engage, for example through transport and support for travel or digital connectivity.

Finally, this chapter demonstrates the importance of nurturing and maintaining weak ties beyond the home, recognising that such connections offer different levels and types of support and belonging, depending on contexts. The potential value of neighbours and neighbouring lies in the seemingly trivial and mundane support rather than in affording them any special or privileged status, and it is relevant to acknowledge that those living with dementia are also neighbours, able to make their own contribution to the social life of neighbourhood places. Nonetheless, neighbouring is for the most part comprised of small, almost inconsequential, acts, and neighbourhoods, however conceptualised and experienced, cannot replace the need for support to deal with structural inequities. Rather, viewing neighbourhoods as relational phenomena offers a useful lens though which to access and understand some of the more overlooked geographies of everyday life with dementia.

Acknowledgements

The authors would like to thank all participants who generously gave their time to the research. The work reported was funded jointly by the Economic and Social Research Council (ESRC) and the National Institute for Health Research (NIHR). The ESRC is part of UK Research and Innovation. The views expressed are those of the authors and not necessarily those of the ESRC or the NIHR This work formed part of the ESRC/NIHR Neighbourhoods and Dementia mixed methods study (https://sites.manchester.ac.uk/neighbourhoods-and-dementia/) and is taken from work programmes 4.

References

Alidoust, S., Bosman, C. and Holden, G. (2018) 'Talking while walking: An investigation of perceived neighbourhood walkability and its implications for the social life of older people', *Journal of Housing and the Built Environment*, 33: 133–50.

Alzheimer's Disease International (2018) *Dementia Friendly Communities: Key Principles* (online), available from: https://www.alz.co.uk/dementia-friendly-communities [Accessed 5 February 2021].

Andrews, G.J., Evans, J. and Wiles, J. (2013) 'Re-spacing and re-placing gerontology: Relationality and affect', *Ageing and Society*, 33(8): 1339–73.

Arup (2019) *Cities Alive: Designing for Age Friendly Communities* [online], available from: https://www.arup.com/perspectives/publications/research/section/cities-alive-designing-for-ageing-communities [Accessed 5 February 2021].

Bartlett, R. and Brannelly, T. (2019) 'On being outdoors: How people with dementia experience and deal with vulnerabilities', *Social Science and Medicine*, DOI:10.1016/j.socscimed.2019.05.041

Baumgartner, D. (1988) *The Moral Order of the Suburb*, New York: Oxford University Press.

Biglieri, S. (2018) 'Implementing dementia-friendly land use planning: An evaluation of current literature and financial implications for greenfield development in suburban Canada', *Planning Practice and Research*, 33(3): 264–90.

Blackman, T. (2006) *Placing Health: Neighbourhood Renewal, Health Improvement and Complexity*, Bristol: Policy Press.

Blackman, T., Mitchell, L., Burton, E., Jenks, M., Parsons, M., Raman, S. and Williams, K. (2003) 'The accessibility of public spaces for people with dementia: A new priority for the "open city"', *Disability and Society*, 18(3): 357–71.

Blackshaw, T. (2010) *Key Concepts in Community Studies*, Los Angeles: Sage.

Blokland, T. (2017) *Community as Urban Practice*, Cambridge: Polity.

Blokland, T. (2003) *Urban Bonds: Social Relationships in an Inner-City Neighbourhood*, Cambridge: Polity.

Bulmer, M. (1986) *Neighbours: The Work of Philip Abrams*, Cambridge: Cambridge University Press.

Campbell, S., Clark, A., Keady, J., Kullberg, A., Manji, K., Rummery, K. and Ward, R. (2019) 'Participatory social network map making with family carers of people living with dementia', *Methodological Innovations* [online], available from: https://doi.org/10.1177/2059799119844445

Cattell, V., Dines, N., Gesler, W. and Curtis, S. (2008) 'Mingling, observing and lingering: Everyday public spaces and their implications for well-being and social relations', *Health and Place*, 14: 544–61.

Charras, K., Eynard, C. and Viatour, G. (2016) 'Use of space and human rights: Planning dementia friendly settings', *Journal of Gerontological Social Work*, 593: 181–204

Clark, A., Campbell, S., Keady, J., Kullberg, A., Manji, A., Rummery, K. and Ward, R. (2020) 'Neighbourhoods as relational places for people living with dementia', *Social Science and Medicine*, DOI:10.1016/j.socscimed.2020.112927

Clarke, C.L., Wilcockson, J., Watson, J., Wilkinson, H., Keyes, S., Kinnaird, L. and Williamson, T. (2020) 'Relational care and co-operative endeavour – Reshaping dementia care through participatory secondary data analysis', *Dementia: The International Journal of Social Research and Practice*, 19(4): 1151–72.

Crow, G., Allan, G. and Summers, M. (2002) 'Neither busybodies nor nobodies: Managing proximity and distance in neighbourly relations', *Sociology*, 36(1): 127–45.

Duggan, S., Blackman, T., Martyr, A. and Van Schaike, P. (2008) 'The impact of early dementia on an outdoor life: A shrinking world?' *Dementia: The International Journal of Social Research and Practice*, 7(2): 191–204.

van Eijk, G. (2012) 'Good neighbours in bad neighbourhoods: Narratives of dissociation and practices of neighbouring in a "problem" place', *Urban Studies*, 49(14): 3009–26.

Emirbayer, M. (1997) 'Manifesto for a relational sociology', *American Journal of Sociology*, 103(2): 281–317.

Hammoud, A., Deriaz, M. and Konstantas, D. (2018) 'Wandering behaviors detection for dementia patients: A survey', 3rd International Conference on Smart and Sustainable Technologies (SpliTech), Split [online], available from: https://ieeexplore.ieee.org/abstract/document/8448329 [Accessed 5 February 2021].

Herbert, C. and Scales, C. (2017) 'Dementia friendly initiatives: A state of the science review', *Dementia: The International Journal of Social Research and Practice*, 15(3): 453–61.

Hydén, L.C. (2017) *Entangled Narratives: Collaborative Storytelling and the Re-Imagining of Dementia: Explorations in Narrative Psychology*, Oxford: Oxford University Press.

Keady, J., Campbell, S., Barnes, H., Ward, R., Li, X., Swarbrick, C., Burrow, S. and Elvish, R. (2012) 'Neighbourhoods and dementia in the health and social care context: A realist review of the literature and implications for UK policy development', *Reviews in Clinical Gerontology*, 22: 150–63.

Kontos, P. and Grigorovich, A. (2018) 'Integrating citizenship, embodiment, and relationality: Towards a reconceptualization of dance and dementia in long-term care', *The Journal of Law, Medicine and Ethics*, 46(3): 717–23.

Kontos, P., Miller, K.L. and Kontos, A. (2017) 'Relational citizenship: Supporting embodied selfhood and relationality in dementia care', *Sociology of Health and Illness*, 39: 182–98.

Lawton, M. (1983) 'Environment and other determinants of well-being in older people', *The Gerontologist*, 23: 349–57.

Lawton, M. and Nahemow, L. (1973) 'Ecology and the aging process', in Eisdorfer, C. and Lawton, M. (eds) *The Psychology of Adult Development and Aging*, Washington DC: American Psychological Association, pp 619–74.

Li, X., Keady, J. and Ward, R. (2021) 'Transforming lived places into the connected neighbourhood: A longitudinal narrative study of five couples where one partner has an early diagnosis of dementia', *Ageing and Society*, 41(3), 605–27.

Lin, Q., Zhang, D., Chen, L., Ni, H. and Zhio, X. (2014) 'Managing elders' wandering behavior using sensors-based solutions: A survey', *International Journal of Gerontology*, 8(2): 49–55.

Macdonald, G. (2019) 'Why person-centred care is not enough: A relational approach to dementia', in Macdonald, G. and Mears, J. (eds) *Dementia as Social Experience: Valuing Life and Care*, Abingdon: Routledge, pp 95–214.

Massey, D. (2005) *For Space*, London: Sage.

Mitchell, L. and Burton, E. (2006) 'Neighbourhoods for life: Designing dementia-friendly outdoor environments', *Quality in Ageing and Older Adults*, 7(1): 26–33.

Mitchell, L., Burton, E., Raman, S., Blackman, T., Jenks, M. and Williams, K. (2003) 'Making the outside world dementia-friendly: Design issues and considerations', *Environment and Planning B: Planning and Design*, 30(4): 605–32.

Odzakovic, E., Hellström, I., Ward, R. and Kullberg, A. (2018) '"Overjoyed that I can go outside": Using walking interviews to learn about the lived experience and meaning of neighbourhood for people living with dementia', *Dementia: The International Journal of Social Research and Practice*, DOI:10.1177/1471301218817453.

Pink, S. (2007) 'Walking with video', *Visual Studies*, 22(3): 240–52.

Poortinga, W. (2012) 'Community resilience and health: The role of bonding, bridging, and linking aspects of social capital', *Health and Place*, 18: 286–95.

Pred, A. (1984) 'Place as a historically contingent process: Structuration and the time-geography of becoming places', *Annals of the Association of American Geographers*, 74(2): 279–97.

Schubert, D. (2000) 'The neighbourhood paradigm: From garden cities to gated communities', in Freestone, R. (ed) *Urban Planning in a Changing World: The Twentieth Century Experience*, London and New York: Routledge, pp 118–38.

Shoval, N., Wahl, H.-W., Auslander, G., Isaacson, M., Oswald, F., Edry, T., Landau, R. and Heinik, J. (2011) 'Use of the global positioning system to measure the out-of-home mobility of older adults with differing cognitive functioning', *Ageing and Society*, 31: 849–69.

Smith, A. (2009) *Ageing in Urban Neighbourhoods: Place Attachment and Social Exclusion*, Bristol: Policy Press.

Sturge, J., Nordin, S., Sussana Patil, D., Jones, A., Légaré, F., Elf, M. and Meijering, L. (2021) 'Features of the social and built environment that contribute to the well-being of people with dementia who live at home: A scoping review', *Health Place*, DOI: 10.1016/j.healthplace.2020.102483

Tampubolon, G., Nazroo, J., Keady, J. and Pendleton, N. (2018) 'Dementia across local districts in England 2014–2015', *International Journal of Geriatric Psychiatry*, 33: 1127–31.

Ward, R., Clark, A., Campbell, S., Graham, B., Kullberg, A., Manji, K., Rummery, K. and Keady, J. (2018) 'The lived neighbourhood: Understanding how people with dementia engage with their local environment', *International Psychogeriatrics*, 30(6): 867–80.

Wettstein, M., Wahl, H.W., Shoval, N., Oswald, F., Voss, E., Seidl, U., Frölich, L., Auslander, G., Heinik, J. and Landau, R. (2015) 'Out-of-home behavior and cognitive impairment in older adults: Findings of the SenTra Project', *Journal of Applied Gerontology*, 34(1): 3–25.

Wiersma, E. and Denton, A. (2016) 'From social network to safety net: Dementia-friendly communities in rural northern Ontario', *Dementia: The International Journal of Social Research and Practice* 15(1): 51–68.

Wigg, J. (2010) 'Liberating the wanderers: Using technology to unlock doors for those living with dementia', *Sociology of Health and Illness*, 32: 288–303.

Wiles, J., Allen, R., Palmer, A., Hayman, K., Keeling, S. and Kerse, N. (2009) 'Older people and their social spaces: A study of well-being and attachment to place in Aotearoa New Zealand', *Social Science and Medicine*, 68: 664–71.

3

Moving house with dementia

Jill Batty

My name is Jill. I married my husband, Dominic, in 1975. He was 46 and I was 29. We had two children in 1976 and 1979. Dominic was a dentist and somewhat eccentric, so we have never been Mr & Mrs Average. He retired in 1996 aged 65. He was diagnosed with Alzheimer's in 2003 and had a diagnosis earlier than most. Perhaps because of his medical training Dominic was aware early on something was not right – as was I. He was initially prescribed Aricept. He stayed on this for a few months but became dizzy and nauseous so stopped taking it. He has taken no medication since then and his dementia has developed relatively slowly. He is now 91. In 2019 we moved to a new house. I didn't tell Dominic about the move as I thought it might distress him. This record is written very much from my perspective and is not necessarily an example of 'good practice' for others to follow. It is simply my account of what it was like for me to move house with a partner who had been living with dementia for 17 years.

One of the joys of living with someone for 45 years is that you get to know each other inside out. I can always tell if Dominic is anxious or uncomfortable. Even if he doesn't voice his feelings to me (and he usually does!) he can become withdrawn and restless. Initially the diagnosis made little difference to our lives. In fact, it was a relief to both of us because it explained Dominic's loss of memory, constant repetitions and change in behaviour. But as the dementia has progressed I feel I have grown in my recognition and ability to deal with what some might perceive to be the gradual slipping away of the man I married.

I immediately joined the Alzheimer's Society and found their fact sheets invaluable. I have always been a great believer in "get help before you need it". As time went on, we went together to a dementia cafe and 'Singing for the Brain'. Dominic used to go alone to an activity group run by the Alzheimer's Society weekly and he also attended alone a course of sessions run by a newly created memory clinic. As his dementia developed Dominic started to attend a day centre one day a week and I paid for a companionship carer (the Lovely Adrian) for four hours a week so I could get out. As time went on I gradually did more and more for Dominic, including all personal care. He was retreating more and more into himself but was not aggressive or difficult. We sang a lot together and he continued to play the piano. I have always felt he is lucky in that I am 17 years younger than him and so can care for him more easily. By 2018 Dominic's physical mobility was deteriorating and, as we lived in a tall house with many stairs, it became apparent we needed to move. We had lived in the same house in Islington for 44 years but, for family reasons and to be near our granddaughter, decided to move to a new neighbourhood south of the river, Dulwich. The distance was about nine miles, but Londoners take the north/south divide very seriously so this was a really big step for us! My friends thought I was bonkers and warned that the change would have a detrimental effect on Dominic. I think they felt it would be confusing for him to be uprooted from home and that he might have difficulty finding his way round the new house. Knowing him better I had no such qualms. I was the mainstay and centre of Dominic's life so, as long as I was with him, I knew he would be fine. I knew he would forget about the old house very quickly and indeed that proved to be the case. It would have been distressing for me had he constantly said he wished we were back in Islington. But I knew we were moving to a house similar in many ways and were taking all our old familiar furniture with us. Before the move I found out about a day centre for him and that there was a local carers' support group. Luckily the Lovely Adrian was to continue weekly visiting which was fantastic – a bit of stability. We were to live on the ground floor of the new house while our son was to live, separately, upstairs.

The move itself was well planned and relatively stress free (the negotiations were a nightmare and took nearly a year but Dominic was blissfully unaware of any problems). The removal men came two days before to pack up so there was very little to do on the day of the move. I arranged for Adrian to be available for as much of the day as we needed him. He collected Dominic and took him to a neighbour's where they had a normal time of singing and lunch. I arranged for two taxis to take us to the new house – one for me and our daughter, and one for Dominic and Adrian. When Dominic and Adrian arrived at the new house they settled in the bedroom as arranged and carried on singing and had more lunch away from the 'chaos' in the rest of the house. After about an hour the removal men left and I felt we were settled enough for Adrian to leave and Dominic to join us in the new kitchen. I feel that Dominic seemed unaware of what was going on. As long as he had normality with him (Adrian or me, singing, food) he was happy. He apparently loved the long taxi ride! He had his own bed with me sleeping in the same room. Only once next day did he ask when we were going back to the other house and I am certain he forgot all about it almost immediately – although typically he remembers his childhood home! I think he had a particularly happy childhood (although he said he never got on with his sister, who was seven years older than him and bossed him about!). His father created two wonderful albums with photos going back to the early 1920s with lots of pictures of the family home. He still spends time looking at them and talks about the lawns that it was his job to cut. He enjoys talking about that house and there seems no need to remind him about the Islington house.

The move has been a great success for us all. Within a few days of moving in I asked my next-door neighbours in for coffee. They told me about Link-Age, a vibrant local charity providing support for older people. Almost immediately we joined their singing group. I could get Dominic there easily on the bus in his wheelchair. Within two weeks of moving and following an assessment by the manager, Dominic started at the day centre I had contacted before the move (they collected him and delivered him back). Initially Dominic went for one day, with Adrian continuing on another day. After about six months Adrian decided to leave caring. He and I had discussed this at length – after all, I had seen him every week for four years so we knew each other well and I understood why he wanted the change. Dominic then went for three days to the day centre. He was always happy to go and indeed regularly played the piano for them there. It is only Covid-19 that has stopped him going now. But the Alzheimer's means he has forgotten he used to go there and is perfectly content at home with me.

Soon after moving in I joined everything I could that interested me – the Dulwich Picture Gallery, the local Picturehouse and the University of the Third Age, through which I have made many acquaintances and one or two good friends. We are lucky to be surrounded by good neighbours although I made a point of getting to know them fairly quickly. The days Dominic was at the day centre gave me some free time. From all the years of caring I have come to recognise that as long as I am happy, then Dominic is contented and relaxed. Our son lives upstairs (although we don't live together) and he is a great support. We all love the new house – it is easier for me and Dominic being on the ground floor and we have a splendid garden. I go to the monthly carers' support group run by the Alzheimer's Society, which has been a helpful source of information and support.

My best friends from 'the North' have all visited on several occasions or we have arranged to meet halfway. I have reassured them that their fears about uprooting Dominic were ill-founded. Thinking back, the move for us was made at the right time. Dominic's dementia was at a point where he did not appear to be very aware of what was happening in the here and now. My son and I spent a lot of time looking for the right house in the right position, and I planned the day of the move very carefully so as not to distress Dominic. Had we moved earlier when he was still going out on his own and would have been more aware of the situation, things might have been more difficult. But importantly I had made enquiries and got things in place for him before we moved. I registered with a GP almost immediately although we had no need to visit as Dominic took no medication. However, the GP is currently referring us for an assessment for a hoist as I fear Dominic will soon become bedbound. We already have a hospital bed and riser chair organised through the local occupational therapist.

When Dominic was diagnosed in 2003 I still felt I was his wife, not his carer. Gradually over the years and with his decline I came to realise I was simply his carer. The advice to carers is always "look after yourself first and foremost because if you go down you are no use to your loved one". I was careful to remember this when preparing for, during and after our move. That is why I made sure I found out about the services and support groups in the new area long before we moved. In so many ways things have been better for us in our new home and I feel we have no reason to move again, whatever the future brings. This may be a bit of the luck of the draw – had we needed to move earlier on in Dominic's dementia, it could well have been distressing and confusing for him, which in turn would have been distressing for me. As it was, his apparent lack of awareness, or at least lack of concern about what was happening, meant that I was never really worried about the effect of the move on him. As long as I was with him, I knew he would he be happy. This left me free and with the energy to concentrate on the practicalities of the move, the advance planning and accessing local services to ensure life continued smoothly. Long may it continue as we move into the end-of-life phase of Dominic's dementia.

4

How do people with dementia manage problematic situations in public spaces?

Anna Brorsson

Introduction

It is now well established that following a diagnosis of dementia, people value being able to continue with their lives and pursue everyday activities, including those performed outside the home, in public space (Öhman and Nygård, 2005; Phinney et al, 2007). In this chapter, public spaces are considered as places outside the home (Brorsson, 2013) and this includes spaces related to (1) retail/consumerism, administration and self-care locations, (2) places for medical care, (3) social, spiritual and cultural places, and (4) places for recreation and physical activities including places for transportation (Margot-Cattin et al, 2019).

Internationally, it is increasingly the case that cities are striving to be 'dementia-friendly' (Lin and Lewis, 2015) or 'age friendly' (WHO, 2007). Yet, public spaces still show deficits that limit activity and restrict the participation of older people and those living with dementia. Moreover, older people in general are sensitive to environmental planning and development; they often bear the consequences, as do people with dementia, of urban planning that has failed to include their needs or perspectives (WHO, 2007). However, there are differences in terms of the use and occupation of public space between individuals with dementia compared to a wider older population. For instance, it has been argued that people with dementia visit a more restricted range of public venues and spaces (Gaber et al, 2019), with associated changes to their social participation, in comparison to non-cognitively impaired older people (Gaber et al, 2020). As such, in order to develop both dementia- and age-friendly societies it is of paramount importance that older people with dementia are included in processes of urban planning, development and commissioning (Phillipson et al, 2018). As the well-established notion states: 'Nothing about us, without us'

(Charlton, 1998), a mantra that has now been adopted by networks of people with dementia. However, to date there has been limited research on how problems in public spaces are experienced by people living with dementia and the strategies and actions they use to meet these situations. The aim of this chapter is therefore to add to our knowledge of how these situations arise and how people living with dementia respond. Such knowledge is vital in fostering a more accessible and usable public domain, providing insights that can inform and guide the direction of future policy and practice.

This chapter is based on a constant comparative analysis (Corbin and Strauss, 2008) of the findings from four studies undertaken by the author (Brorsson et al, 2011, 2013, 2016, 2018). The data from each of the four studies were treated as a discrete dataset and analysed using constant comparative analysis (Corbin and Strauss, 2008). The synthesis of the analysis is presented with new core categories, categories and sub-categories taken from the findings.

A mix of qualitative data collection methods were used in the studies (Brorsson et al, 2011, 2013, 2016, 2018), including semi-structured interviews (Patton, 2002), participant observations (Burgess, 1984), visual methods (Suchar, 1997) and focus group interviews (Kreuger and Casey, 2000) in combination with photo documentation (photos and film sequences) (Harper, 2002). The inclusion criteria were people living with mild to moderate stage dementia, who were independently carrying out everyday activities in public space and living in ordinary housing. In Table 4.1, aim, demographic information and data collection are presented for each of the four included studies.

The complex relationship between person, activity and public space

My interest in environment and accessibility started during my training and subsequent employment as an occupational therapist. The goal in occupational therapy is to enable people to participate in meaningful activities. At the heart of the profession is a commitment to promoting well-being and health though activity (Letts et al, 2003; Christiansen and Townsend, 2004). However, within occupational therapy it has been common to view the environment as a fairly static container in which people exist and perform activities of everyday life (Cutchin, 2004). Underlying theory has been based on the notion of environmental demands and the relative competence of the person in meeting these (Lawton, 1986; Baum and Christiansen, 2005; Kielhofner, 2008). According to this dualistic view, the environment

Table 4.1: Overview of included studies

	Study 1	Study 2	Study 3	Study 4
Aim	To illuminate experiences of accessibility in public space in people with AD, with particular focus on places, situations and activities that they found to be important for daily life.	To discover and describe problematic situations and critical incidents that took place when people with AD performed the ordinary outside-home activity of grocery shopping and how these were met by them.	To identify and examine space characteristics in the space of a grocery shop that may influence how its accessibility is perceived by people with dementia.	To identify problematic situations in crossing at zebra crossings and to identify how people with dementia would understand, interpret and act in these problematic situations.
Informants (n)	n=7	n=6	n=6	n=6
• Female/male	5/2	4/2	6/0	3/3
• Cohabiting/single	3/4	3/3	1/5	3/3
• City centre/suburb	3/4	2/4	1/5	3/3
• Age mean (range)	68.8 (64–80)	69.7 (63–80)	63.6 (57–70)	74.8 (66–86)
• Diagnosis	7×AD	6×AD	5×AD 1×FTD	6×AD
Data collection	In-depth interviews 13 interviews	In-depth interviews and observations 12 interviews 8 observation	Visual methods: 1. photos 2. focus group interviews with photo elicitation 3 photo sessions (372 photos) 2 focus group interviews	Visual methods: 1. film sequences 2. focus groups interviews with film elicitation 3. interviews 22 recordings (1 hr 32 mins) 2 focus group interviews 3 individual interviews

Note: AD = Alzheimer's disease, FTD = Frontotemporal dementia and person are regarded as separate units, but at the same time it has been argued that the environment is a part of the person (Kielhofner, 2008). To deepen our understanding of the complex relationship between the environment (especially public space), activity and the person, a transactional perspective was adopted for this research. The benefit of using this approach is that it allows us to step away from the dualistic view of person–environment, narrowly focused on 'environmental press' and the often fading capacities of the person, and instead to introduce a more holistic and processual approach.

The transactional perspective is based on the theory of action and originates from the philosopher John Dewey, where the focus is upon ongoing transactions between the person and the environment (Cutchin and Dickie, 2012b). In this context, a person's body is viewed as a dynamic process of individual and physical elements (Cutchin and Dickie, 2012a). Taking a holistic view of relations means that entities are considered parts of each other instead of being separate from one another. Further, the places that people transact with are not just physical and material; they include political, cultural and social contexts. Spatial and temporal dimensions are embedded in transactional relations (Cutchin and Dickie, 2012a).

Informed by its origins in occupational therapy, activity is an important concept in the studies described in this chapter and can be regarded as a transaction connecting the person and situations. They are parts of each other; activity can be understood as the glue between the person and environment (Cutchin et al, 2008). The notion of situations originates from symbolic interactionism (Blumer, 1986). A situation is understood to be in a constant state of change and thus when a situation changes a person's actions will also change (Trost and Levin, 2010). Of course, certain situations could be experienced as problematic (Cutchin and Dickie, 2012a). From a transactional perspective, problematic situations are the basis of human action and adaptation, initiating how people coordinate with their environment (Cutchin, 2004).

Another concept used in our discussion is 'place integration', which is based on a combination of the philosophy of John Dewey and geographical theory (Cutchin, 2001) developed by Cuthin (Cutchin, 1999, 2003). Place integration is the ongoing process of creating relative harmony and new meanings in new situations (Cutchin, 1997, 2001). However, this process in not always successful (Aldrich and Cutchin, 2013). People strive to attain the best possible harmony and the process of place integration is ongoing and never complete. In their efforts to establish harmony in situations, people employ actions reflectively,

Figure 4.1: Overview of core category, categories and sub-categories

---

Core category:

An infinite, unstable and challenging process of meeting problematic situations

Categories:

The importance of having access to places and everyday activities in public space to people with dementia

Problematic situations in public space

Vulnerability and the feeling of being exposed in public space

Clutter and crowding

Layout variations

Unpredictable changes

Actions used to maintain access to everyday activities in public space

Use of familiar activities in familiar spaces and places

Avoiding situations leading to new problematic situations

Use of time

Getting help from people

---

which have moral, aesthetic and social qualities (Cutchin, 2004). Drawing upon this notion of a non-linear process has proven to be useful in the generation of understanding of older people's experience of problems in different environments and how they handle these situations (Johansson et al, 2009).

In the following the findings of the four studies (Brorsson et al, 2011, 2013; Brorsson, 2013; Brorsson et al, 2016, 2018) will be presented with core categories, categories and sub-categories (see Figure 4.1).

The importance of having access to places and everyday activities in public space for people with dementia

Having access to everyday activities in public space as long as possible was highly rated for people living with dementia in the context of an awareness of the progressive nature of dementia, and the potential that their ability to access and perform activities outside the home could diminish over time (Brorsson et al, 2011).

Numerous places outside the home were considered important to the informants, such as grocery shops (Brorsson et al, 2011, 2013, 2018), pharmacies, hospitals, care centres and banks (Brorsson et al,

2011). On the whole informants preferred these places to be in the neighbourhood, and within walking distance from home; many had abandoned places that required other means of transport to get there (Brorsson et al, 2011). Places further away were also often perceived as unfamiliar and hence avoided on that basis (Brorsson et al, 2011, 2013). In other words, the activity radii of many of the research informants had become smaller regarding activities and places visited independently and therefore they preferred to frequent places within walking distance from home (Brorsson et al, 2011).

It was crucial for persons living with dementia to have access to different places in order to perform everyday activities (Brorsson et al, 2011, 2013, 2016, 2018). Such access enabled people to feel a sense of independence and social inclusion as active citizens (Brorsson et al, 2011). Activities performed in public space often took on greater importance and significance than they had before their diagnosis. This was exemplified by the experience of grocery shopping, where research informants had come to appreciate the variety of opportunities it offered, such as social contact, exercise by walking to and from the shop, and naturally the actual grocery shopping itself (Brorsson et al, 2011).

Problematic situations in public space

Vulnerability and the feeling of being exposed in public space

While performing everyday activities in public space, people living with dementia could face a variety of challenges. Problematic situations could arise due to difficulties related to staying in control and being focused (Brorsson et al, 2011, 2016). Feelings of vulnerability and of being exposed were also common (Brorsson et al, 2011) and were related to finding one's way while outdoors, for example going to and from the grocery shop (Brorsson et al, 2013, 2018) as well as difficulties inside the grocery shop and in paying (Brorsson et al, 2018). This was described by one informant 'Yes ... I'm very afraid of someone taking my handbag, my keys, and other such things. That's what I worry about the most' (Brorsson et al, 2011, p 593). They also reported feelings of vulnerability when being out late at night, when they experienced difficulties in finding their way and not feeling safe (Brorsson et al, 2011). Informants were aware of the potential of being exposed as having dementia if they could not manage everyday technologies such as self-service checkouts in the shops, cash machines, computers or communication with answering machines (Brorsson et al, 2011). This resulted in a broader sense of social exclusion, as expressed by one informant who commented 'We are actually excluded from a big part of society today, that we are' (Brorsson et al, 2011, p 594). Participants also reported feeling vulnerable as pedestrians, having to interact with different traffic sitatuions, such as short time intervals of traffic lights, resulting in their having difficulties in reaching the other side of the street and sometimes resulting in being stuck at traffic islands in the middle of the road, with cars passing close by on either side (Brorsson et al, 2013, 2016).

People living with dementia could, from time to time, experience mental fatigue when performing activities in public space and this tiredness could influence perceived vulnerability and how they experienced accessibility in public space that day. However, such mental fatigue could be experienced even before entering public space because of all the necessary preparatory actions in the home (Brorsson et al, 2011). Fatigue could also be triggered by difficulties in coping with successive challenges in public spaces and managing all the layers of problematic situations, and in addition the threat or fear of being exposed as struggling to cope (Brorsson et al, 2016).

Potentially stressful situations were a pervasive factor when performing activities in public space and influenced the experience of vulnerability. Stress could hit informants very quickly when they experienced an unexpectedly problematic situation and influence how they tackled that situation. Before their diagnosis of dementia, people recalled acting in a calm way in comparable situations. This was illustrated by one informant who commented 'When I get stressed I can't really handle it and then I act very oddly', they continued 'because I get stressed and then I can't remember anything. Everything seems to disappear' (Brorsson et al, 2018, p 9).

Many informants reported difficulties in discriminating between and making sense of different events or conditions in public spaces and these situations were often unpredictable. These situations could be related to heavy traffic (Brorsson et al, 2016) and noise for example from cars, people and everyday technologies such as refrigerators in grocery shops (Brorsson et al, 2011, 2013, 2016, 2018). Problems with blocking out noise in public space were highlighted: 'So sounds are very, very tough and tiring ...There is no filter anymore' (Brorsson et al, 2011, p 296).

Clutter and crowding

Clutter and crowding could impact upon the accessibility of a space or setting. Too much clutter and overcrowding made it difficult for the informants to concentrate and to stay in focus (Brorsson et al, 2016).

This was revealed through analysis of photographs from a grocery shop and then discussing them in relation to people's experiences. An overload of products and in-store information led the informants to experience the shop as less accessible and less usable. The feeling of clutter and crowding influenced their ability to stay in focus, leading to increased stress levels when doing grocery shopping (Brorsson et al, 2018). This was described by one informant: 'I think that they've brought out too many products when they stand them along the wall like this. There's so much anyway, it seems odd to bring them out when there's already so much' (Brorsson et al, 2018, p 8).

Visuo-perceptive difficulties sometimes added to the confusion and stress caused by clutter and crowding inside the shop. For example, mirrors created an illusion of more products at the vegetable stands and some informants reported trying to pick vegetables from the mirrors. Visual difficulties were also related to glass walls and doors that created problems in distinguishing the walls and doors from the room itself. Some informants reported walking right into the glass walls and doors and hurting themselves (Brorsson et al, 2018). One conversation we had about glass doors included these comments: 'I have banged into it like that. Not that anything got broken ... but that's luck'; 'It's lucky for your head!' (Brorsson et al, 2018, p 10).

Overcrowding could also be related to people in public space for example at the zebra crossing on pavements (Brorsson et al, 2011, 2013, 2016), in the grocery shop (Brorsson et al, 2011, 2013, 2018) or caused by the density and volume of traffic on the road (Brorsson et al, 2016). Furthermore, crowding could also relate to there being a great quantity of products and information all over the store, which made it challenging for the informants to find and choose the intended product (Brorsson, 2013; Brorsson et al, 2018).

Crowding was even sometimes experienced in the home when a lot of items were visible and ready to be used. This situation could lead to difficulties in finding items required for performing activities in public space, such as a wallet and keys (Brorsson et al, 2013).

Layout variations

A logical layout was an important characteristic for enhancing accessibility of public spaces for people living with dementia. Shops and other venues became less accessible when the layout was altered, sometimes unexpectedly, for example when shop managers rearranged products in the grocery shop (Brorsson et al, 2013, 2018). By contrast, at home, people had the possibility to organise the layout of domestic spaces and maintain order, and thereby maintain a feeling of being in control (Brorsson et al, 2013).

Variation between layouts could also prove problematic, for example when these differed between grocery shops and when the grocery shop included different services such as pharmacies or post offices (Brorsson et al, 2016). Also, when the layout was changed within an already familiar shop, it became even more difficult for people to find their way through the shop or locate what they needed (Brorsson et al, 2013, 2018). Therefore, many participants reported that they chose to shop in the same shop, once it had become familiar, and much preferred the layout and organisation of the space to remain unchanged (Brorsson et al, 2013, 2018).

A complex layout could also be experienced as problematic. This could be related to a zebra crossing that had several traffic lights, traffic islands or traffic lanes that offered many options for crossing the street. Such layouts were sometimes experienced as confusing, even overwhelming, and as a result people sought out crossings that were simpler, such as those with one traffic light and one lane in each direction (Brorsson et al, 2016).

Unpredictable changes

Unpredictable changes in public space could create a range of problematic situations and influenced how people living with dementia experienced access to particular venues or settings and their performance of everyday activities. Because of unpredictable or unexpected changes some informants reported difficulties in finding their way, for example from their home, to and from the grocery shop, and in the grocery shop itself (Brorsson et al, 2011, 2013, 2018). Landmarks in public space often proved vitally important in finding the way and when changes were made to a landmark they relied on, or it disappeared altogether, they could more easily get lost as a result. Examples of this include a house that had been repainted in a new colour, and a public art statue that had been removed (Brorsson et al, 2011).

Changes could also be related to noise, crowding and tempo in public space and traffic density when such aspects were in a constant state of change and could be difficult to predict in advance (Brorsson et al, 2011, 2013, 2016, 2018). Controlling and maintaining order became difficult for people living with dementia due to unpredictable changes. A familiar place could therefore randomly change and become unfamiliar, compromising the person's experience of accessibility.

Actions used to maintain access to everyday activities in public space

In the following, characteristics of the actions used to meet problematic situations will be described.

Use of familiar activities in familiar spaces and places

Performing familiar activities in familiar settings was an important means to maintain a degree of independence, when out and about (Brorsson et al, 2011). Many informants reported frequenting familiar shops within walking distance from home (Brorsson et al, 2013), and they used road crossings that were familiar and not too complex, for example zebra crossings with traffic lights (Brorsson et al, 2016). To find a product in the shop, they often bought the same brands because the packages were recognisable and therefore familiar (Brorsson, 2013). To find their way in the shop they took the same route, thus maintaining their familiarity with its layout (Brorsson et al, 2018). However, familiar spaces and places could often change and thus the informants could experience a new problematic situation when, for example, a landmark had changed, or a familiar brand had new packaging. This demonstrated that it is of great importance to people living with dementia to have the opportunity to continue to perform familiar daily activities in familiar places in order to maintain their connection to different public spaces. This was achieved through daily routines and habits (Brorsson, 2013).

Avoiding situations leading to new problematic situations

People living with dementia understood that the actions they used in order to meet problematic situations could be unsuccessful and that a new challenge could occur as a result. Consequently, they made efforts to avoid these situations. One example was the use of a shopping list as a reminder for knowing what to buy. However, if the shopping list was forgotten at home, the person could experience problems in remembering what to buy and this could result in going shopping several times in one day (Brorsson et al, 2013). In this way a challenging situation or lapse in memory could reverberate throughout the day, leading to further challenges. This situation was shared by one informant: 'Then I have written a shopping list but I have forgotten that. I don't know how I can forget so much' (Brorsson et al, 2013, p 295).

People also carefully planned how to pay for their groceries when payment itself could lead to new problematic situations, as they had difficulties in counting money or using credit cards. Some were concerned about using the self-service checkouts and worried about whether the ordinary counter desk would be open at the grocery shop (Brorsson et al, 2013, 2018). The informants avoided crowding in shops, on pavements and at zebra crossings, when they knew from previous experience that these conditions could all lead to new problematic situations. For instance, some participants found themselves stepping into the road to avoid crowding on the pavement (Brorsson et al, 2011, 2013, 2016, 2018).

Use of time

There was also a temporal aspect to people's actions for managing problematic situations. For instance, some informants planned what time of day to perform activities, avoiding the crowding in the shop in the late afternoon. Hence, many preferred to shop in the morning (Brorsson et al, 2011, 2018). Some informants preferred to wait some time when arriving at the zebra crossing to avoid the crowding of pedestrians (Brorsson et al, 2016). However, this strategy could create unexpected challenges such as when they no longer had time to cross safely when the traffic light turned red. Activities in the late afternoon or evening were commonly performed together with relatives or friends as this was the time of day when public space was often perceived to be less accessible. It was also very common for informants to plan to have a lot of time at their disposal when performing activities, particularly if stress influenced them negatively and could hit them very quickly (Brorsson et al, 2013, 2018). For example, when going grocery shopping, they gave themselves plenty of time to avoid stressful situations arising (Brorsson et al, 2013).

Getting help from people

Getting help from people was one way of tackling problematic situations. For example, people would commonly ask for help if they could not find certain products in the grocery shop (Brorsson et al, 2013) or they got lost when out and about (Brorsson et al, 2011, 2013). Some informants asked staff or other shoppers for help, but others avoided these situations as they did not want to reveal their diagnoses (Brorsson et al, 2013, 2018). A number of people revealed that they were sensitive and selective regarding whom to ask for help.

Interestingly, some asked women rather than men and did not ask people who appeared to be in a hurry, or people who did not seem to live in the area. The informants also relied on help from cashiers when they had difficulties in counting money; they could hand over their money to the cashier to take the right amount (Brorsson et al, 2013). Another non-verbal approach to getting help was in trying to establish eye contact with drivers when crossing the street by waving a hand or raising their canes in the air, to let them cross (Brorsson et al, 2016).

An infinite, unstable and challenging process of meeting problematic situations

In this chapter different activities performed by people with dementia have been studied, including grocery shopping, being a pedestrian and doing activities in general in public space. In these situations, the complex relationship between the person, activity and public space (environment) was described by using a transactional perspective and is further developed in the core finding: *An infinite, unstable and challenging process of meeting problematic situations.* This core finding summarises the fluid and processual dimension to a person's relationship to public space when living with dementia and underlines the effortful nature of time spent outdoors in public settings.

As might be expected, we found that people with dementia must unavoidably relate to a diversity of situations when performing activities in public space, many of which may be unforeseen. Normally, they would meet the more routine and everyday situations with well-rehearsed actions or approaches that are performed in an unthinking and habitual way and thereby were not experienced as problematic. However, people with dementia experienced many situations in public space that for one reason or another had become problematic in comparison with their experience prior to diagnosis. I have shown here that a problematic situation as a whole often contained multiple layers of difficulty that posed challenges. When performing activities outside the home, in public space, people therefore had to relate to the numerous layers of a problematic situation, as public space was in a state of constant flux, with much happening at the same time (Brorsson, 2013).

In each of the studies considered here, different layers of problematic situations were identified (see Table 4.2). This could be associated with an array of different, often sensory, factors such as visuo–perceptive difficulties, intrusive auditory stimuli (from people talking, to noise from cars and humming sounds from refrigerators in the grocery

Table 4.2: Problematic situations as a whole, layers of problematic situations and actions used to meet layers of problematic situations

Problematic situations as whole – preparations in home	Actions used to meet layers of problematic situations
Layers of problematic situations	• Bring a note of what to bring, buy and do.
• Remember what to bring and what activity to be performed in public space.	• Keep strict order in home to find objects.
• Clutter of objects, many objects ready to be used.	

Problematic situations as whole – in general, public space	Actions used to meet layers of problematic situations
• Interpretation of signs, timetables and maps.	• Avoid stressful situations.
• Locate signs.	• Regular daily or weekly, space–time patterns in shopping. Take walks in the same places.
• Crowded places with fast tempo and noise.	• Do fewer demanding activities.
• Find the way in late afternoon and evening.	• Do activities together with friends or relatives.
• Replacement of service personnel with everyday technologies (computers, self-service checkouts).	• Do activities within an activity radius of home.
• Communications with answering machines and following different steps.	

Problematic situations as whole – finding the way	Actions used to meet layers of problematic situations
• Change of landmarks.	• Choose small shop within walking distance from home.
• Reconstruction of houses and streets.	• Shop with friends or relatives.
	• Use transportation for old and disabled when going far away from home.
	• Use street signs.
	• Ask people for help.

Problematic situations as whole – crowding of pedestrians	Actions used to meet layers of problematic situations
• Crowding at the zebra crossing and pavements.	• Avoid crowding by walking around it.
• Chaotic pattern of pedestrians at zebra crossings.	• Wait some time to avoid the rush at green light at zebra crossing.
• Pedestrians do things simultaneously when crossing the zebra crossing.	

Problematic situations as whole – crossing a street

- Unsure if cars would stop or not.
- Drivers not using indicators for turning.
- Gaps between vehicles.
- Direction of vehicles.
- Closeness of cars.
- Cyclist and drivers ignoring traffic rules.
- Discriminate and understand different road markings.
- Discriminate marks at zebra crossing covered with snow.
- Discriminate things from each other at the crossing when the colour is the same (grey).
- Stumble on objects such as traffic islands.
- Discriminate silent vehicles.
- Discriminate sounds and what sounds to direct their attention to.

Actions used to meet layers of problematic situations

- Walk longer distance to avoid complex layout of zebra crossing.
- Use of traffic lights as a reminder and security precaution.
- Use of zebra crossing with or without traffic lights.
- Wait until no cars are coming down the road.
- Walk with relatives.
- Be a cautious pedestrian.
- Signal to drivers.
- Follow the flow of other pedestrians.

Problematic situations as whole – grocery shopping

- Influenced by people being stressed in the shop, for example the cashier.
- Packing groceries.
- Count money.
- Use of self-service checkout.
- Use of credit card.
- Remember security code for credit card.
- Choose the right membership card.
- Get through when aisles are crowded.
- Many different services in grocery shop.
- Locations of products.
- Illogical layout of checkouts such as card reader and change machinery for coins.
- Objects and information all over the shop.
- Clutter and crowding.
- Mirrors, glass doors and walls creating visual illusions.
- Background music and noise.

Actions used to meet layers of problematic situations

- Search for object in an unstructured way.
- Walk around in the shop to find the intended product.
- Use of signs to find objects.
- Take one's time when searching.
- Talk to oneself.
- Observe illustrations on products.
- Buy the same familiar brand of products.
- Importance of pre-understating of layouts of shops.
- Walk the same routes in shop.
- Go along the walls of the shop.
- Prefer small shop, but at the same time broad aisles.
- Hand over money to cashier.
- Pay with a large-denomination bill.
- Avoid credit cards.
- Sign receipt when using credit card.
- Hand over membership cards to cashier to choose the right one.

shop), as well as other factors such as weather conditions, complex layouts at zebra crossings and in grocery shops. These different layers of challenging conditions transacted and could create a problematic situation as a whole. The fluid, changeable nature of public spaces meant that one problematic situation in a particular season, day or moment could involve one set of challenges but another day it may present another set of layers, thereby creating a totally new situation. The insight here is that places are rarely experienced as fixed and stable and this changeable nature of public venues and settings poses particular challenges for anyone living with dementia. These findings demonstrate how the person and public space are in constant interplay (Brorsson, 2013).

A person with dementia can experience cumulative challenges, and as these build up in the course of the day they may lead to mental fatigue, which in turn can further compromise the accessibility of public spaces. Yet, these layers of problematic situations could prove less problematic another day when the person had fewer problems with preparations in the home before entering public space and consequently experienced less fatigue (Brorsson et al, 2011, 2013, 2016). This reasoning has been further developed in Brorsson et al, 2011, where a transactional perspective was used to explain the core finding: *Accessibility as a constantly changing experience*. This core finding underlines that there is a continuous interaction between the public space and the person and therefore accessibility is experienced as a continuously changing set of conditions. This insight was elaborated with the metaphor of a kaleidoscope representing the essence of people's experience of public spaces when living with dementia. In the kaleidoscope, small loose objects, which represent the different layers of a situation, alter as the kaleidoscope is turned. As the changes occur, a completely new design or pattern emerges, representing the new experience of accessibility.

Meeting layers of problematic situations with different actions was, for the informants, an infinite, unstable and challenging process. The actions they employed were characterised by creativity, open-ended reflections and drawing upon previous experience, all of which underlined their own agentive and adaptive responses to the situations they found themselves in. People living with dementia used different strategies to meet problematic situations, often having to adapt in the moment to unexpected twists and turns. The actions to meet these situations could seldom be predicted in advance because circumstances in public space changed continuously and the ever-changing relationship between the environment and person varied, sometimes from moment to moment. The research participants sometimes struggled to coordinate when multiple tasks or actions were required simultaneously (Brorsson et al, 2016). Hence, the challenging process of finding strategies to meet layers of problematic situations was never stable and often unpredictable and could even generate new or subsequent challenges.

Conclusion

By using a transactional perspective to understand problems that people with dementia experience when performing activities in publics space, and noting their actions in meeting these situations, I have begun to outline key considerations for creating an age and dementia-friendly society. The different ways that people living with dementia tackle problematic situations, as described here, are certainly recognisable to many people and are not exclusively related to living with dementia. I have shown here that when using a transactional perspective, we can generate useful knowledge about how people engage with their social and physical environment. The findings may highlight the complexity of creating cognitively accessible and usable public spaces but also point to ways that such spaces can be altered and adapted that can measurably impact on the day-to-day experiences of people with dementia. For instance, based on the studies described in this chapter, guidance for shop managers has been developed on how to create a dementia-friendly grocery shop (MFDSE, 2016). Overall, I have demonstrated the value of drawing upon the lived experience of people with dementia as a framework for creating more inclusive neighbourhoods and in so doing have highlighted the need for change to our urban and public spaces.

References

Aldrich, R. and Cutchin, M. (2013) 'Dewey's concept of embodiment, growth, and occupation: Extended bases for transactional perspective', in Dickie, V. and Cutchin, M. (eds) *Transactional Perspective on Occupation*, New York: Springer, pp 13–24.

Baum, C. M. and Christiansen, C. H. (2005) 'Person-environment-occupation-performance: An occupation-based framework for practice', in Christiansen, C. H., Baum, C. M. and Bass-Haugen, J. (eds) *Occupational Therapy. Performance, Participation, and Well-being*, 3rd edn, Thorofare, NJ: SLACK, pp 242–66.

Blumer, H. (1986) *Symbolic interactionism: Perspective and Method*, Berkeley, University of California Press.

Brorsson, A. (2013) *Access to everyday activities in public space, views of people with dementia*, PhD thesis, Karolinska Institutet.

Brorsson, A., Öhman, A., Cutchin, M. and Nygård, L. (2013) 'Managing critical incidents in grocery shopping by community-living people with Alzheimer's disease', *Scandinavian Journal of Occupational Therapy*, 20: 292–301, https://doi.org/10.3109/11038128.2012.752031

Brorsson, A., Öhman, A., Lundberg, S., Cutchin, M.P. and Nygård, L. (2018) 'How accessible are grocery shops for people with dementia? A qualitative study using photo documentation and focus group interviews', *Dementia*, 1471301218808591, https://doi.org/10.1177/1471301218808591

Brorsson, A., Öhman, A., Lundberg, S. and Nygård, L. (2011) 'Accessibility in public space as perceived by people with Alzheimer's disease', *Dementia*, 10: 587–602, https://doi.org/10.1177/1471301211415314

Brorsson, A., Öhman, A., Lundberg, S. and Nygård, L. (2016) 'Being a pedestrian with dementia: A qualitative study using photo documentation and focus group interviews', *Dementia*, 15: 1124–40, https://doi.org/10.1177/1471301214555406

Burgess, R. (1984) *In the Field: An Introduction to Field Research*, London and New York: Routledge.

Charlton, J.I. (1998) *Nothing About Us Without Us: Disability Oppression and Empowerment*, Berkeley: University of California Press.

Christiansen, C. and Townsend, E. (2004) *Introduction to Occupation. The Art and Science of Living*, Upper Saddle River: Prentice Hall.

Corbin, J. and Strauss, A. (2008) *Basics of Qualitative Research*, Thousand Oaks: Sage Publications, Inc.

Cutchin, M., Aldrich, R., Bailliard, A. and Coppola, S. (2008) 'Action theories for occupational science: The contribution of Dewey and Bourdieu', *Journal of Occupational Science*, 15: 157–65, https://doi.org/10.1080/14427591.2008.9686625

Cutchin, M. and Dickie, V. (2012a) 'Transactional perspectives on occupation: An introduction and rational', in Cutchin, M. and Dickie, V. (eds) *Transactional Perspective on Occupation*, New York: Springer, pp 1–12.

Cutchin, M. and Dickie, V. (2012b) 'Transactionalism: Occupational science and the pragmatic attitude', in Whiteford, G. and Hocking, C. (eds) *Occupational Science, Society, Inclusion, Participation*, Oxford: Blackwell Publishing Ltd, pp 23–37.

Cutchin, M.P. (1997) 'Community and self: Concepts for rural physician integration and retention', *Social Science & Medicine*, 44: 1661–74, https://doi.org/10.1016/S0277-9536(96)00275-4

Cutchin, M.P. (1999) 'Qualitative explorations in health geography: Using pragmatism and related concepts as guides', *The Professional Geographer*, 51: 265–74, https://doi.org/10.1111/0033-0124.00163

Cutchin, M.P. (2001) 'Deweyan integration: Moving beyond place attachment in elderly migration theory', *International Journal of Aging & Human Development*, 52: 29–44, https://doi.org/10.2190/af2d-a0t4-q14c-1rtw

Cutchin, M.P. (2003) 'The process of mediated aging-in-place: A theoretically and empirically based model', *Social Science & Medicine*, 57: 1077–90, https://doi.org/10.1016/s0277-9536(02)00486-0

Cutchin, M. (2004) 'Using Deweyan philosophy to rename and reframe adaptation-to-environment', *The American Journal of Occupational Therapy*, 58(3): 303–12, https://doi.org/10.5014/ajot.58.3.303

Gaber, S.N., Nygård, L., Brorsson, A., Kottorp, A. and Malinowsky, C. (2019) 'Everyday technologies and public space participation among people with and without dementia', *Canadian Journal of Occupational Therapy*, 86(5): 000841741983776–411, https://doi.org/10.1177/0008417419837764

Gaber, S.N., Nygård, L., Brorsson, A., Kottorp, A., Charlesworth, G., Wallcook, S. and Malinowsky, C. (2020) 'Social participation in relation to technology use and social deprivation: A mixed methods study among older people with and without dementia', *International Journal of Environmental Research and Public Health*, 17: 4022, https://doi.org/10.3390/ijerph17114022

Harper, D. (2002) 'Talking about pictures: A case for photo elicitation', *Visual Studies*, 17: 13–26.

Johansson, K., Borell, L. and Lilja, M. (2009) 'Older persons' navigation through the service system towards home modification resources', *Scandinavian Journal of Occupational Therapy*, 16: 227–37, https://doi.org/10.3109/11038120802684307

Kielhofner, G. (2008) *Model of Human Occupation: Theory and Application*, 4th edn, Philadelphia: Lippincott Williams & Wilkins.

Kreuger, R. and Casey, M. (2000) *Focus Groups: A Practical Guide for Applied Research*, Thousand Oaks: Sage Publications, Inc.

Lawton, M.P. (1986) *Environment and Aging*, Albany: Center for the Study of Aging.

Letts, L., Rigby, P. and Stewart, D. (2003) *Using Environments to Enable Occupational Performance*, Thorofare: SLACK Inc.

Lin, S.-Y. and Lewis F.M. (2015) 'Dementia friendly, dementia capable, and dementia positive: Concepts to prepare for the future', *The Gerontologist*, 55(2): 237–44, https://doi.org/10.1093/geront/gnu122

Margot-Cattin, I., Kuhne, N., Kottorp, A., Cutchin, M., Öhman, A. and Nygård, L. (2019) 'Development of a questionnaire to evaluate out-of-home participation for people with Dementia', *The American Journal of Occupational Therapy*, 73(1): 7301205030p1–7301205030p10, https://doi.org/10.5014/ajot.2019.027144

MFDSE (2016) 'Det ska vara lätt och handla' [It should be easy to do grocery shopping] (online), 28 November, available from: https://www.youtube.com/watch?v=0Tluj9VQmsM

Patton, M.Q. (2002) *Qualitative Research and Evaluation Methods*, Thousand Oaks: Sage.

Phillipson, L., Hall, D., Cridland, E., Fleming, R., Brennan-Horley, C., Guggisberg, N., Frost, D. and Hasan, H. (2018) 'Involvement of people with dementia in raising awareness and changing attitudes in a dementia friendly community pilot project', *Dementia*, 18: 2679–94, https://doi.org/10.1177/1471301218754455

Phinney, A., Chaudhury, H. and O'Connor, D.L. (2007) 'Doing as much as I can do: The meaning of activity for people with dementia', *Aging & Mental Health*, 11: 384–93, https://doi.org/10.1080/13607860601086470

Suchar, C. (1997) 'Grounding visual sociology research in shooting scripts', *Qualitative Sociology*, 20(1), 33–55, https://doi.org/10.1023/A:1024712230783

Trost, J. and Levin, I. (2010) *Att förstå vardagen med ett symbolisk interaktionistiskt perspektiv*, Pzkal: Studentlitteratur AB, Lund.

WHO (2007) *Global Age-friendly Cities: A Guide*, available from: http://www.who.int/ageing/publications/Global_age_friendly_cities_Guide_English.pdf [Accessed 7 May 2018].

5

Making and maintaining neighbourhood connections when living alone with dementia

*Elzana Odzakovic, Agneta Kullberg, Ingrid Hellström,
Andrew Clark, Sarah Campbell, Kainde Manji, Kirstein
Rummery, John Keady and Richard Ward*

Introduction

This chapter draws on qualitative research using participatory methods to explore the experience of people with dementia who live alone. Drawing on data gathered in Sweden and the UK, the chapter highlights the distinct challenges of living alone with dementia and explores the different ways that people remain connected to neighbourhood places. We argue that the invisibility of such experiences to dementia policy and strategies (which typically assume the presence of a cohabiting carer or household member to provide support) needs to be addressed if dementia-friendly initiatives are to be truly inclusive.

Demographic projections show that the number of people living in single households will continue to increase steadily in many western and northern European countries and that older women are the fastest-growing section of the single householder population (Sundström et al, 2016; United Nations, 2017). The ageing population living alone in Europe also includes an increasing proportion of people with dementia (Prescop et al, 1999; Gaymu and Springer, 2010; Prince et al, 2015). In Canada, France, Germany, the UK and Sweden, between one third and one half of the population of people with dementia residing in a neighbourhood context live in single households (Ebly et al, 1999; Nourhashemi et al, 2005; Alzheimer's Society, 2013; Eichler et al, 2016; Odzakovic et al, 2019). Despite this increase in single householders with dementia, there is currently limited awareness of the particular challenges associated with living alone with dementia, even within emerging discourses and practices associated with dementia-friendly communities (Alzheimer's Society, 2013; Age UK, 2018; Odzakovic et al, 2018). As such, there is a danger that the creation of 'dementia-friendly' communities, and especially those based on communities of place, may rest upon a series of normative assumptions about dementia and about the relational context of people living with the condition.

Evidence from service-oriented research shows that people with dementia who live alone are more prone to (unplanned) hospitalisation (Ennis et al, 2014); are at greater risk of malnutrition (Nourhashemi et al, 2005); are likely to be admitted to long-term care at an earlier point in their journey with dementia (Yaffe et al, 2002); are often less well connected to formal services (Webber et al, 1994); and lack the advocacy of a co-resident carer (Eichler et al, 2016). However, to date, little is known of the lived experience of neighbourhood for people with dementia who live alone, including how they manage possible isolation, limit the risk of loneliness, and remain socially connected outside the home.

Background

Neighbourhoods, ageing and dementia

In recent years, policy consensus has emerged concerning the benefits of empowering people living with dementia to remain active participants in their local community as part of a shift away from institutionalisation (World Health Organization, 2017; Alzheimer's Disease International, 2018). In England, Scotland and Sweden the respective governments have formulated national plans and strategies for dementia with an emphasis on social inclusion and quality of life, and, to varying degrees, have supported a commitment to foster dementia-friendly communities (Department of Health, 2012; Department of Health and Social Care, 2015; The Scottish Government, 2017; Socialdepartementet, 2018). A dementia-friendly community has been defined as 'a place or culture in which people with dementia and their carers are empowered, supported and included in society, understand their rights and recognize their full potential' (Alzheimer's Disease International, 2016, p 10).

A key factor in sustaining quality of life and well-being in later life is through access to the social environment surrounding the home, a sphere that can be defined in many western cultures as 'the neighbourhood' (Wiles, 2005; Bowling, 2008). While there are many definitions of what a neighbourhood is, this chapter focuses particularly on the social environment and the ways in which locally situated relationships and contacts are developed and maintained and alter over time for people living alone with dementia. In this context, it is argued that neighbourhood conditions play a significant role in mediating connectivity and social inclusion/exclusion (Milligan et al, 2004; Age UK, 2018).

As social networks constrict, this can lead to loneliness, with attendant implications for both mental and physical health (Larson, 1990; Burger, 1995; Victor et al, 2009). There is increasing evidence that the risk of social isolation is compounded by the onset of illness or disability (Tomaka et al, 2006; Hilberink et al, 2017) and after the onset of dementia (Fratiglioni et al, 2000). It is helpful to distinguish between isolation, which is the objectively defined situation of being alone with an absence of social interactions and often linked to being confined at home (Larson, 1990; Burger, 1995), and the more subjectively defined condition of loneliness (Perlman and Peplau, 1981).

Previous research on people living alone with dementia at home has tended to focus narrowly on support in the home, where 'community dwelling' is often equated with support aimed at enabling individuals to 'manage at home' (Lehman et al, 2010; Miranda-Castillo et al, 2010; Alzheimer's Society, 2013). There is also evidence that those who live alone have more restricted opportunities for sociability (Duane et al, 2011). However, a growing body of research has begun to explore how people with dementia interact with their wider neighbourhood (Blackman et al, 2007; Duggan et al, 2008; Keady et al, 2012; Phinney et al, 2016; Kelson et al, 2017; Brorsson et al, 2018; Ward et al, 2018; Clark et al, 2020). For instance, evidence suggests that regular walks in/through the neighbourhood support different types of interaction and social encounters for people living with dementia (Odzakovic et al, 2018; Ward et al, 2018). Yet, little research has focused specifically on those living alone with the condition in a neighbourhood context.

To date, less emphasis has been given to understanding the broader social circumstances or revealing how people with dementia themselves experience living alone with a progressive condition. The purpose of this chapter is therefore to explore how people in this situation establish and maintain connections and relationships in a neighbourhood context, and asks what support, if any, they receive in so doing. More broadly, the chapter aims to contribute to debate on care at home and the development of 'dementia-friendly communities' (Alzheimer's Society, 2013).

Methods

Walking interviews, social network mapping, home tours and semi-structured interviews

This chapter draws on data collected from a work package of the ESRC/NIHR funded Neighbourhoods and Dementia programme (See also Chapters 2 and 7 in this book). The Neighbourhoods: Our People, Our Places (N:OPOP) research project used a mix of qualitative data collection methods (Morse and Niehaus, 2009) including walking interviews (Carpiano, 2009; Clark and Emmel, 2010; Clark, 2017; Kullberg and Odzakovic, 2017), social network mapping (Emmel and Clark, 2009; Clark, 2017; Campbell et al, 2019) and home tours, which drew on Pink's (2009) 'walking with video method' across three fieldsites in England, Scotland and Sweden. An overview of data collection is presented in Figure 5.1 which shows the slightly differing order and approach between the UK and Swedish sites.

Recruitment

The recruitment of participants aimed to include people living with dementia (those with a diagnosis and those providing care and support). Ethical approval was obtained from the NHS Health and Social Care Research Ethics Committee in the UK and the Regional Ethical Review Board in Linköping (the county of Östergötland, Sweden). In total, 127 participants were selected to participate across the three fieldsites and, of those, 67 were participants with a diagnosis of dementia and 60 were primary carers. We selected participants from the total of 127 participants based on the following inclusion criteria: living alone (without a cohabiting partner/children/next of kin), not sharing their living accommodation with others (that is, a one-person household). All the participants were community dwelling and able to give oral and/or written informed consent.

A process consent approach (Dewing, 2008) was followed with regular reminders about the research. The first contact with potential participants was by letter and/or telephone call. The researchers asked to return to conduct subsequent interviews after a period of 8–12 months (Figure 5.1) as an opportunity to explore any changes to the participants' situation over time. The participants and/or caregivers decided the time and place for the interviews, and none of the participants withdrew during the interviews.

Some of the participants only took part in one round of interviews (this was often due to a decline in health or having moved on from

Figure 5.1: Overview of how data collection was undertaken in the three fieldsites

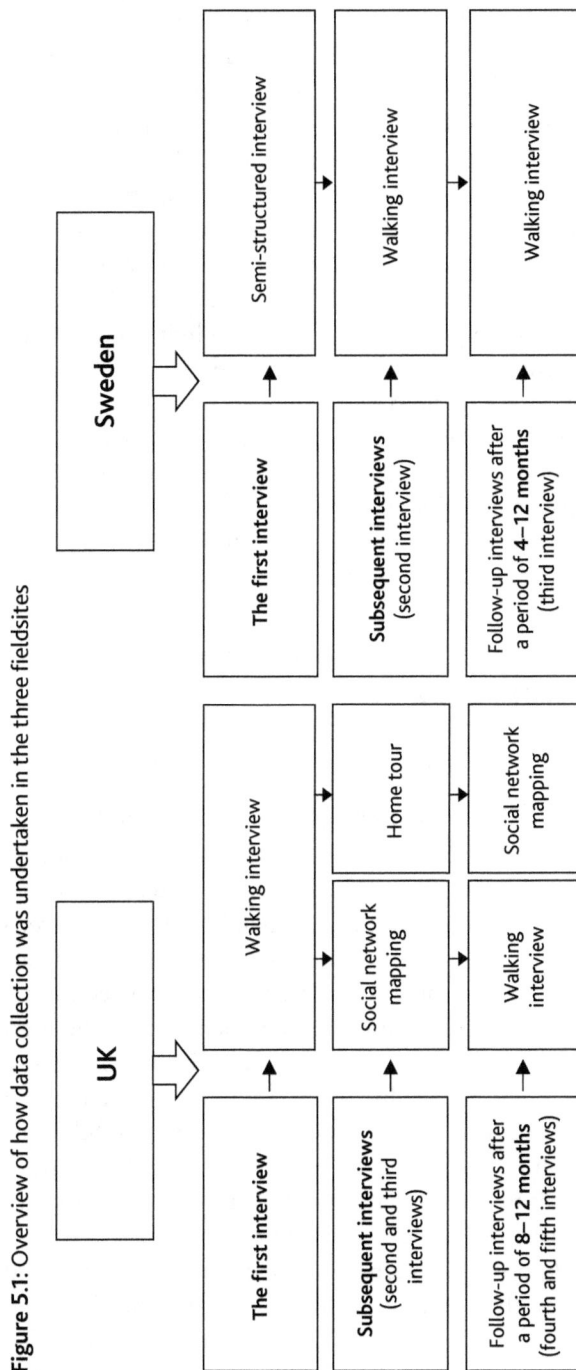

their original address); others agreed to participate in a follow-up interview (Table 5.1). In total, 14 community-dwelling people living alone with dementia participated in at least one of the multiple data collection methods in the study. The participants ranged in age from 62 to 88 years; 11 were women and three were men (see Table 5.1). Each had a diagnosis of dementia although some chose not to or were unable to reveal the specific type of dementia. Some participants were managing at home without formal support, whereas others had regular visits from different dementia practitioners, including home care services. Previous research has looked at solitude or loneliness primarily from the perspective of women living alone with dementia within a domestic context and has not explored the wider world of neighbourhoods that hold social opportunities for people living alone with dementia as active citizens (deWitt et al, 2009, 2010; Frazer et al, 2011; Lloyd and Stirling, 2011; Svanström and Johansson Sundler, 2015). Our data provide unique insights into the lived experiences of both women and men living alone with dementia and their desire to sustain social connections in their neighbourhood.

The neighbourhood experiences of people living alone with dementia

Working hard to stay connected

Participants spoke of their efforts to stay connected, often in the face of social losses as contact with friends and sometimes even family decreased after a diagnosis of dementia. Many reported that some close relationships with family, friends and neighbours had evolved over many years and withstood the impact of the diagnosis. For instance, ties with some close family members were reported to have been sustained much as before the onset of dementia; the resilience of these connections highlighted their value to those involved. Maintaining a relationship with family, and especially with children, also helped to facilitate broader connections to friends and neighbours. Children often gave ongoing prompts and reminders, made bookings for events and carried out research into local social opportunities that were passed on to their parents. In this way, social networks were collectively managed even when this support was offered from a distance. Kathleen and Margaret outlined how their family facilitated broader social connections and events: "The family were here in this room and it was a lovely sunny afternoon. And loads of people came. They stayed the night. We had a real party. They ended up having a glass of wine and I made the beds

Table 5.1: Participants' characteristics (some characteristics altered to preserve anonymity)

Pseudonym	Age (rounded to nearest 5) (years)	Gender	Dwelling type and location	Years in the dwelling (at time of the interview)	Marital status	Former (primary) occupation	Interview type (year when the interview took place)	Country of residence
Anna	80	F	Flat, town	5 or fewer	Widowed	Manual	Semi-structured (2016), walking (2016)	Sweden
Alma	70	F	Flat, town	5 or fewer	Unmarried	Manual	Semi-structured (2016)	Sweden
Bodil	90	F	Detached house, rural	Over 50	Widowed	Health and social care	Semi-structured (2016)	Sweden
Cecilia	80	F	Flat, town	5 or fewer	Widowed	Manual	Semi-structured (2013), walking (2013)	Sweden
Doris	80	F	Flat, town	Unknown	Widowed	Clerical/administration	Semi-structured (2016)	Sweden
Fanny	85	F	Flat, town	Between 6 and 10	Widowed	Health and social care	Semi-structured (2014), walking (2014)	Sweden

(continued)

Table 5.1: Participants' characteristics (some characteristics altered to preserve anonymity) (continued)

Pseudonym	Age (rounded to nearest 5) (years)	Gender	Dwelling type and location	Years in the dwelling (at time of the interview)	Marital status	Former (primary) occupation	Interview type (year when the interview took place)	Country of residence
Harold	80	M	Cottage, rural	Between 11 and 20	Widowed	Agricultural	Walking (2015), home tour (2016), social network mapping (2015)	UK
Ingvar	60	M	Flat, town	Over 20	Unmarried	Creative industries	Semi-structured (2014), walking (2014)	Sweden
June	80	F	Two-storey house, suburb	Over 30	Widowed	Home maker	Home tour (2015), social network mapping (2015)	UK
Kathleen	85	F	Terraced house, urban	Over 30	Widowed	Home maker	Walking (2016), home tour (2016)	UK
Margaret	80	F	Detached house, town	Between 11 and 20	Widow	Clerical/ administration	Walking (2017), social network mapping (2017)	UK
Mike	65	M	Flat, town	Between 6 and 10	Unmarried	Armed forces	Walking (2017), social network mapping (2017)	UK

(continued)

Table 5.1: Participants' characteristics (some characteristics altered to preserve anonymity) (continued)

Pseudonym	Age (rounded to nearest 5) (years)	Gender	Dwelling type and location	Years in the dwelling (at time of the interview)	Marital status	Former (primary) occupation	Interview type (year when the interview took place)	Country of residence
Sandra	90	F	Flat, urban	Over 20	Widowed	Manual	Walking (2016), social network mapping (2016), home tour (2016)	UK
Åsa	80	F	Flat, town	Over 20	Widow	Clerical/administration	Semi-structured (2016)	Sweden

up" (Kathleen, UK); "It is really because my children go to the church, then [vicar] visits me at home as often as he can" (Margaret, UK).

Those without children reported focusing their efforts on a niece or nephew, a circle of friends or sometimes just one or two key social contacts. These relationships played a similarly crucial role in maintaining wider neighbourhood connections. Participants also described efforts to maintain existing relationships and to establish new ones. In some of our discussions, we identified a longing to engage in daily social interactions in the neighbourhood as a means of maintaining a degree of continuity in everyday life. For instance, June worked hard to keep up relationships with her friends: "I can still go out like ... Well, my friends come. We go to [local venue] and we sometimes have a pub lunch" (June, UK).

People highlighted the significance of having a friend they could chat with and who looked out for them, which provided a sense of reassurance. Sometimes, 'weak ties' (Granovetter, 1973), such as shopkeepers or other local residents, were helpful just in knowing that someone was looking out for them. However, participants also faced the challenge of seeking out and establishing new contacts and, in some cases, rebuilding their networks. Some interviewees reported wanting to participate in different clubs or meeting places to avoid being alone. Doris (Sweden) shared how her experience of living alone could sometimes tip over into a sense of loneliness, a feeling that had become more acute since her diagnosis of dementia. Doris was a 79-year-old woman, living in an apartment in an urban area. She received support from the municipality-run home care service and had an alarm installed at the front door after an incident when she had left her apartment in the middle of night. After the alarm was installed, Doris told us that she had begun to feel like a prisoner in her own home and had been increasingly neglected by her neighbours:

> 'So, if I were to go and open the door, then they [staff from home care services] notice it. If some good friend calls and says "we are going to go to the cinema tonight," would you like to come along? No, I can't, as I'm a prisoner in my own home.' (Doris, Sweden)

Before her dementia, Doris had a group of friends that she socialised with, but post diagnosis, as she noticed herself forgetting things and sometimes repeating her questions, she found herself increasingly excluded from her social circle:

'I had a group of friends that I joined many years ago. On one occasion, we met up to have a chat with coffee and cake, then they said "should we go over to [venue for the next meet-up]"? Well, I said "where is this place then?" "Don't you know!" Those words, cut right through me. I really don't have any friends here.' (Doris, Sweden)

It was not only Doris who recounted stigmatising social experiences such as this. Ingvar and Cecilia (Sweden) both had experiences of friendships that had fallen away after their diagnosis. Ingvar reflected:"When you get sick no matter what it is ... then friends disappear. Especially, after [being diagnosed with] Alzheimer's" (Ingvar, Sweden).

There was a lack of social awareness regarding what a dementia diagnosis means, but also as these accounts reveal, a lack of acceptance and even compassion, which led to exclusion from social networks over time. Loss of social connections was a feature of most people's post-diagnostic experience, although it was not necessarily interpreted as linked to dementia. For instance, Fanny (Sweden) ascribed the dwindling number of visitors to her home to her age, rather than as a response to her having dementia: "One does not have that many guests, when one gets to this age."

Not everyone had thriving local connections; for instance, we spoke to some people who hardly knew their neighbours and who felt ambivalent about reaching out to such physically proximate but socially more distant connections. Some participants noted that contact with neighbours was limited to sharing the newspaper or to a brief chat in the staircase of their apartment block, but the regularity of such brief encounters over time helped to maintain their sense of connection: "This [neighbour] right over, I do not have much contact with. But the other neighbour usually comes in and wants to know how I'm feeling each day. They are all old neighbours from way back" (Åsa, Sweden).

For others, neighbours provided a low but consistent level of daily support, and this expectation or practice of supportive neighbouring was revealed both in the UK and Sweden. Some reported that their neighbours visited daily just to chat, often without being invited, or called them on the telephone to hear their voice. For others, their neighbours were a more latent source of support that they knew could be relied upon when most needed. For instance, Margaret (UK) reported that her neighbours visited her almost daily, and they also had her daughter's number in case of emergency: "They've got [daughter's] phone number and she's got theirs, but we've never used it yet."

Some participants made regular forays outdoors where there were good chances of more spontaneous encounters and described how they would seek out these popular spaces within their neighbourhood in the hope of a chance encounter, though always during daylight hours. Such places included parks, pubs or cafes and often led to opportunistic encounters with 'regulars' or staff, as Mike (UK) noted about a member of staff at a cafe that he visited daily to drink his morning coffee: "He always has a chat, and he's quite funny at times." In Sweden, there were fewer such neighbourhood-based meeting places, so opportunities for spontaneous encounters were more limited due to the cultural tradition of meeting people outdoors. Getting to know the neighbours or participating in social activities with them was often not deemed a social necessity for many Swedes, which may indicate a broader cultural trait (Ehn, 1996). However, participants revealed various plans and strategies to increase the chances of social interaction in their neighbourhood. This could simply involve taking a walk or carefully selecting where they sat. These strategies supported a sense of inclusion and neighbourhood participation, as outlined by Anna and Fanny: "This summer was too long, then it [seating area in neighbourhood] almost becomes a small meeting point for pensioners. It's our pleasure, we count cars here. I can sit here for a while and sometimes there's nobody to talk to, sometimes there is someone that I can talk with" (Anna, Sweden); "Then one always meets someone one can talk to … when I am out sometimes, and there are [usually] a few people around" (Fanny, Sweden).

As Fanny and Anna indicate, seeking out or making arrangements for spontaneous encounters in the neighbourhood result in new ways to connect with other people and lay the foundations for networks that they would hope to sustain. Despite the differences between the fieldsites, people clearly took pleasure from and invested real effort in maintaining the social networks and relationships of which they were a part. Using different approaches and types of activity was important for people to find new contacts and connections. This leads to questions about how well such efforts were recognised and supported by formal service providers.

Befriending by organisations and facilitated friendship

A number of community organisations and service providers offered regular weekly activities, which the research participants looked forward to. In the UK these were primarily, though not always, led and organised by third sector and charitable groups, whereas in Sweden that support more likely came from the public sector, mainly the local municipality (county council). For many people living alone this support represented a central aspect of their social contact. Home care visits provided an opening for sociability and opportunities for exchange of news and events. For some participants a visit to a voluntary organisation or service provider opened up a social world where they could meet others with the same condition. In this way service providers played the role of 'friendship facilitators' (Ward et al, 2012), creating connections between people living with dementia that could evolve into supportive and close affiliations. The activities on offer were also perceived as good for their health and well-being: "I go to a group that [my son] ... knew the fella that ran it ... I was only there last week. They had a dancing session last week when I went. It is good for your brain, and they're all very friendly" (Margaret, UK).

The volunteers and professionals working within these organisations and local hubs were sometimes described by participants as friends rather than being seen as workers, and the overall atmosphere was described as familiar, comfortable and notably free of stigma. As such, these local venues represented a safe space within the proximate neighbourhood. Crucially, these were spaces that provided opportunities for peer support and more informal camaraderie. Some interviewees indicated that these third sector organisations were the first point of contact for support if anything were to happen to them. For instance, Mike had experienced long spells of unemployment and ill-health. After being diagnosed with dementia he revealed how a support worker from a charitable organisation had encouraged him to attend an activity group that created social opportunities for him at a time when he had felt cut off and increasingly depressed: "I found out about it when I got my diagnosis. They gave me a leaflet and gave me a number to ring. Linda from [charity] came and took me to the club that is run by [the organisation]. They are a really important part of my life now" (Mike, UK).

Interviews conducted in the Swedish fieldsite did not reveal any voluntary/third sector organisations (or designated link workers) involved in the support of people with dementia living alone in the community; the infrastructure for community-based dementia care differs from the UK in this respect. In Sweden municipality-run day care centres served as places where the participants could meet others and participate in different activities during the week. Social activities included sports and exercise classes, and opportunities for eating lunch together. For Doris the day care centre offered a degree of respite from the isolation of life at home: "I'm happy about [day care centre] because it has saved me. I was terribly alone a lot and I can honestly say the day care centre was what saved me" (Doris, Sweden).

The befriending role of third sector organisations and other service providers offered people a focus for social activities and membership of a network that was free of the stigma they perceived and experienced in some other public venues and social events. There were some notable differences between the UK and Swedish fieldsites in terms of which sector and type of organisation took responsibility for coordination and day-to-day running of these neighbourhood hubs. In Sweden there were few indications of engagement by volunteers in the area where we undertook the research, or any real signs of wider involvement of local businesses, retailers or venues such as cafes. Indeed, any noticeable shift towards a more diversified 'mixed economy' of community-based support is yet to establish itself in Sweden compared with the UK. Instead, the municipalities (local county councils) in Sweden took responsibility for day care provision and any other meeting places that people living alone with dementia might frequent. In Sweden's welfare system, home care is available to all citizens irrespective of income, based on an assessment of an individual's needs (Rostgaard and Szebehely, 2012). However, an income-graded fee for the care applies; those on a low income (about one third) do not pay any fee, but this can differ between the municipalities. By contrast, in England and Scotland, there was clear evidence of public sector services having receded, with voluntary/third sector groups serving as the primary source of support and connection within the community. However, irrespective of the nature of the organisations involved, people were clear that the support they received was an important buffer against potential isolation.

The quiet neighbourhood atmosphere

The third theme concerns the neighbourhood atmosphere, particularly the quiet periods when others were at work or school/college. During these times the neighbourhood could feel quite deserted. Participants also reflected on how the tone and atmosphere of a particular neighbourhood evolved more gradually as people moved on and families grew up and moved out. Cecilia shared her experience of a quietening atmosphere after a number of local children, whom she had enjoyed watching and listening to as they played in the street, moved away from her neighbourhood. Every day Cecilia had sat on her sofa in the kitchen, looking out through the window at the children playing outside, and this had proved a restorative experience after a heart attack:

> 'There were many immigrant children on the street playing in the summer. They were so lovely to look at, how they were playing. Then one day I just said: where did all the kids go? I miss the kids! Now it's so quiet that you just wish for the sound of other people.' (Cecilia, Sweden)

For some, a quiet neighbourhood atmosphere was experienced as anything but relaxing or peaceful; participants discussed feelings of insecurity during times when there were no people in sight. This underlined how just seeing people outside provided a degree of neighbourhood connection but also perhaps how it more deeply reinforced a sense of neighbourhood identity. Those who lived alone described taking steps to seek out places where they knew that they would see people walking or moving around, even if these were complete strangers. This underlines the importance of public space as a way of mitigating the quietness of residential areas. The windows and/or balcony were also essential to being able to keep a visual link to a wider world beyond the home. For Kathleen, the window offered a view over her enclosed garden. She could see the cat sitting under the tree or when the postman and her carers came to visit. The window maintained her sense of connection to the world outside and offered opportunities to witness the spatio-temporal changes near home. She noted that her well-being was often lifted through an emotional connection to the neighbourhood outside her window (Coleman and Kearns, 2015; Musselwhite, 2018). Both Kathleen and Alma shared how their windows enabled them to feel connected to life outside, offering a temporary release from domestic confinement, and decreasing their sense of solitude: "I love the window; it gives me a feeling of freedom. I'm not closed in" (Kathleen, UK); "Look what a nice view I have. And I can see everyone who goes to the day care centre. But I can also see those who are walking and shopping, it may seem a bit curious" (Alma, Sweden).

For Sandra, her television provided a means to break the silence during periods of quiet and inactivity in the neighbourhood, especially during holidays, which posed a particular challenge for those left behind in the city: "Oh, it's deathly quiet. It's too quiet, sometimes, because I forget to turn the telly down a bit, and ... of course, because folk go on holiday and you miss them" (Sandra, UK). Even if Sandra, and others in her position, did not actually watch the television, the sound provided background noise that prevented the silence becoming oppressive. Different people coped with living on their own in different ways, but many noted how their sense of solitude and isolation was compounded when a quiet atmosphere descended on the local area. During such times, people reported seeking out activity and movement, and gravitating towards areas they knew would offer opportunities for sociability.

Changing social connections

Much has been written previously about the loss of social connections and gradually shrinking networks as people age, and there is some indication that this experience intensifies in the fall-out from illness or disability in later life (Duggan et al, 2008). Evidence from our research project ostensibly supports this pattern of social losses for many people living with dementia, and it was clear from our discussions with participants that stigma was often perceived to play a pivotal role. However, a particular message from our research is that people with dementia are by no means passive in the face of these losses, taking action to redress the situation, which we would argue needs to be both recognised and better supported by those who provide neighbourhood-based services. Importantly, solitude (as distinct from loneliness or isolation) was found to be a position of choice actively sought out by some participants. Thus, both Ingvar and Harold shared similar perspectives on solitude as a freedom they wished to maintain: "In a way I'm quite asocial as well and here's deathly quiet. But it's good for me ... In my writing, you live with ... with the people in the novel so to speak ... I do" (Ingvar, Sweden); "Yeah, I'm kind of my own buddy. I'm really quite home based" (Harold, UK).

However, some shared experiences where solitude shaded into feelings of loneliness, compounded by the death of a partner, family members or close friends. They wanted to establish new relationships: "I'd love to have someone in my life but how do I go about making that happen? It would be so nice to have someone who came home to me. But I'm just lonely, and I feel as if I can't do anything about it" (Bodil, Sweden).

Some participants felt compelled to take action to tackle an encroaching sense of loneliness but were often not adequately supported to do so. Our interviews underline that greater knowledge and awareness of the particular challenges faced by people living alone with dementia is required, both in social policy but also in frontline practice and service delivery such as health and social care professionals working in primary health care and home care services. While various dementia-friendly community initiatives have the potential to provide support for the increasing number of people with dementia who live alone in the neighbourhood, more needs to be done. Otherwise, there is a risk that a narrow conceptualisation of dementia, and homogenising assumptions about the situation of people living with the condition, may lead to the creation of neighbourhoods that are experienced as exclusionary for many people with dementia who are outside of normative family support structures.

Conclusion

In a recent guide to developing dementia-friendly communities issued by Alzheimer's Disease International (2016), there is only one sentence that refers directly to people living alone with dementia. This indicates that anyone with dementia living as a single householder remains largely unacknowledged in policies concerning dementia-friendly communities, and that specific action needs to be taken to ensure their voices are heard. This chapter has provided insight into the experiences of those living alone with dementia in neighbourhood settings. While stigma undoubtedly influences potential isolation, the participants were not passive in response to their situation. Those we spoke to employed a variety of strategies to facilitate interactions with others and to feel some sense of connection – from attending social events or clubs, to seeking out fairly fleeting encounters in public spaces, or even just acknowledging passers-by from their windows. We have shown that neighbourhoods can enhance or reduce the chances of interaction for people living alone with dementia according to the spatio-temporal rhythms of the day (people at work during the day), or the season (people going away for the summer) or when neighbours move away. The research also shows the importance of weak ties that enable a sense of social connection – and weak ties (by definition) are not 'deep' but are clearly still crucial to establishing social relationships in the neighbourhood. Ultimately, we have shown that the dementia-friendly communities agenda, and other place-based forms of policy and interventions for dementia, need to anticipate and actively support the diversity of relational conditions in which people are embedded. Beyond commonplace assumptions that living alone equates to isolation for anyone with cognitive impairment, we have outlined a far more nuanced and diverse set of experiences.

References

Age UK (2018) *All the Lonely People: Loneliness in Later Life*, London: Age UK. Available from: https://www.ageuk.org.uk/globalassets/age-uk/documents/reports-and-publications/reports-and-briefings/loneliness/loneliness-report.pdf

Alzheimer's Disease International (2016) *Dementia Friendly Communities: Global Development*, London: Alzheimer's Disease International. Available from: https://www.alz.co.uk/adi/pdf/dfc-developments.pdf

Alzheimer's Disease International (2018) *From Plan to Impact, Progress Towards Targets of the Global Action Plan on Dementia*, London: Alzheimer's Disease International. Available from: https://www.alz.co.uk/adi/pdf/from-plan-to-impact-2018.pdf

Alzheimer's Society (2013) *Dementia 2013: The Hidden Voice of Loneliness*, London: Alzheimer's Society. Available from: https://www.alzheimers.org.uk/sites/default/files/migrate/downloads/dementia_2013_the_hidden_voice_of_loneliness.pdf

Blackman, T., Van Schaik, P. and Martyr, A. (2007) 'Outdoor environments for people with dementia: An exploratory study using virtual reality', *Ageing & Society*, 27: 811–25.

Bowling, A. (2008) 'Enhancing later life: How older people perceive active ageing?' *Aging & Mental Health*, 12: 293–301.

Brorsson, A., Ohman, A., Lundberg, S., Cutchin, M. and Nygard, L. (2018) 'How accessible are grocery shops for people with dementia? A qualitative study using photo documentation and focus group interviews', *Dementia*, 19(6): 1872–88.

Burger, J.M. (1995) 'Individual differences in preference for solitude', *Journal of Research in Personality*, 29: 85–108.

Campbell, S., Clark, A., Keady, J., Kullberg, A., Manji, K., Rummery, K. and Ward, R. (2019) 'Participatory social network map making with family carers of people living with dementia', *Methodological Innovations*, 12: 1–12.

Carpiano, R.M. (2009) 'Come take a walk with me: The "go-along" interview as a novel method for studying the implications of place for health and well-being', *Health & Place*, 15: 263–72.

Clark, A. (2017) 'Seeing real life? Working with the visual to understand landscapes of community', *International Review of Qualitative Research*, 10: 190–210.

Clark, A., Campbell, S., Keady, J., Kullberg, A., Manji, K., Rummery, K. and Ward, R. (2020) 'Neighbourhoods as relational places for people living with dementia', *Social Science & Medicine*, 252, https://doi.org/10.1016/j.socscimed.2020.112927

Clark, A. and Emmel, N. (2010) *Using Walking Interviews. Methods Toolkit (ESRC/Realities Node)*, Manchester: University of Manchester.

Coleman, T. and Kearns, R. (2015) 'The role of bluespaces in experiencing place, aging and wellbeing: Insights from Waiheke Island, New Zealand', *Health & Place*, 35: 206–17.

Department of Health (2012) *Prime Minister's Challenge on Dementia. Delivering Major Improvements in Dementia Care and Research by 2015*, London: Department of Health. Available from: https://assets. publishing.service.gov.uk/government/uploads/system/uploads/ attachment_data/file/215101/dh_133176.pdf

Department of Health and Social Care (2015) *Prime Minister's Challenge on Dementia 2020*, London: Department of Health. Available from: https:// www.gov.uk/government/publications/prime-ministers-challenge- on-dementia-2020/prime-ministers-challenge-on-dementia-2020

Dewing, J. (2008) 'Process consent and research with older persons living with dementia', *Research Ethics Review*, 4: 59–64.

deWitt, L., Ploeg, J. and Black, M. (2009) 'Living on the threshold: The spatial experience of living alone with dementia', *Dementia*, 8(2): 263–91.

deWitt, L., Ploeg, J. and Black, M. (2010) 'Living alone with dementia: An interpretive phenomenological study with older women', *Journal of Advanced Nursing*, 66: 1698–707.

Duane, F., Brasher, K. and Koch, S. (2011) 'Living alone with dementia', *Dementia*, 12: 123–36.

Duggan, S., Blackman, T., Martyr, A. and Van Schaik, P. (2008) 'The impact of early dementia on outdoor life. A "shrinking world"?' *Dementia*, 7: 191–204.

Ebly, E.M., Hogan, D.B. and Rockwood, K. (1999) 'Living alone with dementia', *Dementia and Geriatric Cognitive Disorders*, 10: 541–48.

Ehn, S. (1996) *Familj och grannar i byggd miljö*, Stockholm: KTH [in Swedish].

Eichler, T., Hoffmann, W., Hertel, J., Richter, S., Wucherer, D., Michalowsky, B., Dreier, A. and Thyrian, J.R. (2016) 'Living alone with dementia: Prevalence, correlates and the utilization of health and nursing care services', *Journal of Alzheimer's Disease*, 52: 619–29.

Emmel, N. and Clark, A. (2009) *The Methods Used in Connected Lives: Investigating Networks, Neighbourhoods and Communities*, ESRC National Centre for Research Methods, NCRM Working Paper Series 06/09 2009.

Ennis, S.K., Larson, E.B., Grothaus, L., Helfrich, C.D., Balch, S. and Phelan, E.A. (2014) 'Association of living alone and hospitalization among community-dwelling elders with and without dementia', *Journal of General Internal Medicine*, 29: 1451–9.

Fratiglioni, L., Wang, H.X., Ericsson, K., Maytan, M. and Winblad, B. (2000) 'Influence of social network on occurrence of dementia: A community-based longitudinal study', *The Lancet*, 15: 1315–19.

Frazer, S.M., Oyebode, J.R. and Cleary, A. (2011) 'How older women who live alone with dementia make sense of their experiences: An interpretative phenomenological analysis', *Dementia*, 11: 677–93.

Gaymu, J. and Springer, S. (2010) 'Living conditions and life satisfaction of older Europeans living alone: A gender and cross-country analysis', *Ageing & Society*, 30: 1153–75.

Granovetter, M.S. (1973) 'The strength of weak ties', *American Journal of Sociology*, 78: 1360–80.

Hilberink, S.R., van der Slot, W.M.A. and Klem, M. (2017) 'Health and participation problems in older adults with long-term disability', *Disability and Health Journal*, 10: 361–6.

Keady, J., Campbell, S., Barnes, H., Ward, R., Li, X., Swarbrick, C., Burrow, S. and Elvish, R. (2012) 'Neighbourhoods and dementia in the health and social care context: A realist review of the literature and implications for UK policy development', *Reviews in Clinical Gerontology*, 22: 150–63.

Kelson, E., Phinney, A. and Lowry, G. (2017) 'Social citizenship, public art and dementia: Walking the urban waterfront with Paul's Club', *Cogent Arts & Humanities*, 4: 1–17.

Kullberg, A. and Odzakovic, E. (2017) 'Walking interviews as a research method with people living with dementia in their local community', in Keady, J., Hyden, L.C., Johnson, A. and Swarbrick, C. (eds), *Social Research Methods in Dementia Studies: Inclusion and Innovation (Routledge Advances in Research Methods)*, London: Routledge, pp 23–37.

Larson, R.W. (1990) 'The solitary side of life: An examination of the time people spend alone from childhood to old age', *Developmental Review*, 10: 155–83.

Lehman, S.W., Black, B.S., Shore, A., Kasper, J. and Rabins, P.V. (2010) 'Living alone with dementia: Lack of awareness adds to functional and cognitive vulnerabilities', *International Psychogeriatrics*, 22: 778–84.

Lloyd, B.T. and Stirling, C. (2011) 'Ambiguous gain: Uncertain benefits of service use for dementia carers', *Sociology of Health & Illness*, 33: 899–913.

Milligan, C., Gatrell, A. and Bingley, A. (2004) ' "Cultivating health": Therapeutic landscapes and older people in northern England', *Social Science & Medicine*, 58: 1781–93.

Miranda-Castillo, C., Woods, B. and Orrell, M. (2010) 'People with dementia living alone: What are their needs and what kind of support are they receiving?' *International Psychogeriatrics*, 22: 607–17.

Morse, J.M. and Niehaus, L. (2009) *Mixed Methods Design: Principles and Procedures*, Walnut Creek: Left Coast Press.

Musselwhite, C.B.A. (2018) 'The importance of a room with a view for older people with limited mobility', *Quality in Ageing and Older Adults*, 19: 273–85.

Nourhashemi, F., Amouyal-Barkate, K., Gillette-Guyonnet, S., Cantet, C., Vellas, C. and REAL.FR Group (2005) 'Living alone with Alzheimer's disease: Cross-sectional and longitudinal analysis in the REAL.FR Study', *Journal of Nutrition, Health & Aging*, 9: 117–20.

Odzakovic, E., Hellström, I., Ward, R. and Kullberg, A. (2018) ' "Overjoyed that I can go outside": Using walking interviews to learn about the lived experience and meaning of neighbourhood for people living with dementia', *Dementia*, DOI: 10.1177/1471301218817453

Odzakovic, E., Hydén, L.C., Festin, K. and Kullberg, A. (2019) 'People diagnosed with dementia in Sweden: What type of home care services and housing are they granted? A cross-sectional study', *Scandinavian Journal of Public Health*, 47: 229–39.

Perlman, D. and Peplau, L.A. (1981) 'Toward a social psychology of loneliness', in Gilmour, R. and Duck, S. (eds) *Personal Relationships 3: Personal Relationships in Disorder*, London: Academic Press, pp 31–56.

Phinney, A., Kelson, E., Baumbusch, J., O'Connor, D. and Purves, B. (2016) 'Walking in the neighbourhood: Performing social citizenship in dementia', *Dementia*, 15: 381–94.

Pink, S. (2009) *Doing Sensory Ethnography*, London: Sage.

Prescop, K.L., Dodge, H.H., Morycz, R.K., Schulz, R.M. and Ganguli, M. (1999) 'Elders with dementia living in the community with and without caregivers: An epidemiological study', *International Psychogeriatrics* 11: 235–50.

Prince, M., Wimo, A., Guerchet, M., Ali, G.C., Wu, Y.T. and Prina, M. (2015) *World Alzheimer Report 2015: The Global Impact of Dementia*, London: Alzheimer's Disease International. Available from: https://www.alz.co.uk/research/WorldAlzheimerReport2015.pdf

Rostgaard, T. and Szebehely, M. (2012) 'Changing policies, changing patterns of care: Danish and Swedish home care at the crossroads', *European Journal of Ageing*, 9: 101–9.

Socialdepartementet (2018) Nationell strategi för omsorg om personer med demenssjukdom [National Strategy for Care of People with Dementia]. Available from: https://www.regeringen.se/49bcce/contentas-sets/a36c33ecd30e4adb854c48b96a2b83bb/nationell-strategi-for-demenssjukdom.pdf [in Swedish].

Sundström, A., Westerlund, O. and Kotyrlo, E. (2016) 'Marital status and risk of dementia: A nationwide population-based prospective study from Sweden', *BMJ Open*, 6: 1–7.

Svanström, R. and Johansson Sundler, A. (2015) 'Gradually losing one's foothold – a fragmented existence when living alone with dementia', *Dementia*, 14: 145–63.

The Scottish Government (2017) *Scotland's National Dementia Strategy 2017–2020*, Edinburgh: The Scottish Government. Available from: https://www.alzscot.org/assets/0002/6035/Third_Dementia_Strategy.pdf

Tomaka, J., Thompson, S. and Palacios, R. (2006) 'The relation of social isolation, loneliness, and social support to disease outcomes among the elderly', *Journal of Aging and Health*, 18: 359–84.

United Nations (2017) *Living Arrangements of Older Persons: A Report on an Expanded International Dataset*, New York: United Nations. Available from: http://www.un.org/en/development/desa/population/publications/pdf/ageing/LivingArrangements.pdf

Victor, C., Scambler, S. and Bond, J. (2009) 'Social relationships and everyday life', in Victor, C., Scambler, S. and Bond, J. (eds) *The Social World of Older People. Understanding Loneliness and Social Isolation in Later Life*, Maidenhead: Open University Press, pp 81–127.

Ward, R., Clark, A., Campbell, S., Graham, B., Kullberg, A., Manji, K., Rummery, K. and Keady, J. (2018) 'The lived neighbourhood: Understanding how people with dementia engage with their local environment', *International Psychogeriatrics*, 30: 867–880.

Ward, R., Howorth, M., Wilkinson, H., Campbell, S. and Keady, J. (2012) 'Supporting the friendships of people with dementia', *Dementia*, 11: 287–303.

Webber, P.A., Fox, P. and Burnett, D. (1994) 'Living alone with Alzheimer's disease: Effects on health and social service utilization patterns', *The Gerontologist*, 34: 8–14.

Wiles, J. (2005) 'Conceptualizing place in the care of older people: The contributions of geographical gerontology', *International Journal of Older People Nursing*, 14: 100–8.

World Health Organization (2017) *Global Action Plan on the Public Health Response to Dementia 2017–2025*, Geneva: World Health Organization. Available from: https://apps.who.int/iris/bitstream/handle/10665/259615/9789241513487-eng.pdf;jsessionid=BA172 4B44C90C7CCC6D2461EEE325249?sequence=1.

Yaffe, K., Fox, P., Newcomer, R., Sands, L., Lindquist, K., Dane, K. and Covinsky, K.E. (2002) 'Patient and care-giver characteristics and nursing home placement in patients with dementia', *Journal of the American Medical Association*, 287: 2090–7.

6

My neighbourhood, my future ...?

Wendy Mitchell

I was diagnosed with Mixed Dementia, Alzheimer's and Vascular, on 31 July 2014. I may not have much of a short-term memory but that's one date that remains firmly in my ailing brain. At the time I was living happily alone in York and working full time as a non-clinical supervisor in the NHS, teaching Matrons and Sisters how to roster their staff. However, since dementia forced me into retirement I've lived alone, still happily, in a small village in the East Riding of Yorkshire. Being alone here during the pandemic could have been a disaster, but instead has become a triumph over loneliness and has shown me the importance of the people in our neighbourhood. Pre COVID-19, I didn't have time to get to know my village, whereas now, COVID has allowed me the space and time in my life to become and feel connected with those around me.

I moved to my village a year after being diagnosed. The hustle and bustle of York, once adored and embraced by me, was now becoming too loud, too confusing. It was important I found somewhere quieter to call home. My daughter had moved to the village with her partner some time back, so I was used to visiting and this influenced my choice to move here. But what struck me was the friendliness of this neighbourhood. I was a stranger yet people smiled and said hello. I felt comfortable here. So, when my thoughts came to moving, the village seemed the obvious choice. I needed to feel safe, to feel part of a community. I needed to feel I could cope here on my own if my daughter and son-in-law moved away. The village felt right.

Prior to our world changing and the word 'lockdown' entering our vocabulary, I spent most of the week travelling around the country, raising awareness, sowing seeds of knowledge into people's minds about my experience of dementia. I saw it as a gift from dementia, allowing me to retire early, so my gift in return was carving out a new career almost of public speaking and campaigning against the injustices that exist against those of us living with dementia.

Pre dementia I was an extremely private person. Now I've been overtaken by this gregarious 'alien', (a metaphor I use to describe how I've become more outgoing since developing dementia) I need to know people are around me who make me feel safe. Before COVID existed I would be travelling about nearly every day of the week, attending different events, on and off the train, meeting, listening and talking to lots of people.

My motivation was selfish in many ways. My intuition told me that 'doing' was better at stabilising my dementia than simply sitting at home with dementia as my only company. The bonus in all this was that people wanted to listen. They craved to hear the experience of someone with dementia, from someone who could articulate their emotions, their feelings, their experience. What people often didn't appreciate was the amount of effort and time it took to prepare for these talks. It was as though I magically appeared and disappeared. Little did they realise how exhausting it was; how stressful travelling could be; how I tested my ability on every occasion simply to be there. It was then that I started including these thoughts into my talks, after all, my experience wouldn't be real without the reality of the downsides of dementia, of which there are many. But that's all disappeared. Of course, it's disappeared for many, not just me.

Because I travelled about so much pre COVID-19, I didn't really know that many people [in the neighbourhood]. But then this strange alien world entered all our lives and 'lockdown' became a recognised everyday phrase. It was then the relationship with my neighbourhood changed. I live alone, so lockdown was and still is very distressing, particularly the disappearance of my routine, so important for someone with dementia. The new rules to try and remember. Instead of enjoying the rare quiet days where I had me and silence for company, those silent days far outnumber the days when I talk to anyone, creating a strange loneliness ... one like I've never felt before.

I call the village bus 'The NHS on Wheels' as it serves to help people socialise, to catch up on the news, and it should never be lost. The bus service disappeared for a few months and I felt trapped in my village. I love catching our village bus and seeing all the smiles, the cheery hellos and conversations that take place on that short ride into town. However, since COVID and all the new rules, the bus has lost its friendliness as people can't hear what each other's saying with a mask in situ, you can't see the smiley face. But we nod and greet each other. Instead of chattering away, we now sit there in silence. A great shame and a huge social loss.

One positive result came in the shape of our village shop. I'd occasionally use it but not for my daily shopping. That was left until the bus took me into town. Suddenly that was all I had. People living with dementia were left off the vulnerable list for supermarket delivery slots. I couldn't work out how to book a slot anyway. Yes, my daughters would do my shopping for me if I asked, but I see that too as a social activity. It's a chance to talk to people, to see people. The village shop became part of my new routine. I soon got to know everyone. They called me by my name and most importantly, they smiled and asked if I was ok? Suddenly the loneliness started to disappear.

I know I have many Zooms [teleconferences] I could join, but I need to feel people's presence. Zoom has been a lifesaver for so many 'playmates' [my name for other people with dementia] and they want the 'Zoom way' to continue long after COVID for very valid reasons, for those who find travelling difficult or simply don't like travelling, but for me, I adore travelling and the set time to 'have a conversation' instead of the randomness of a few minutes' chat in the street and then a goodbye. But sometimes, just being around people is enough for me; hearing other voices. Unfortunately for me, yet fortunately for so many others, the Zoom world will be with us for a very long time and that makes me sad. I know I'll have to overcome those feelings or I'll miss out on so much, but I also know it would never be my first choice. Technological connection has been a lifeline for many, but for me, it's caused frustration and each time has emphasised my need for human contact face to face.

Nature around me suddenly became so important. Whereas pre COVID, I'd be travelling about via train to experience new environments now all I had to explore was my neighbourhood. I started looking for public footpaths to venture down, for walks I'd not done before; discovering new environments right on my doorstep, ones I never knew existed. Suddenly COVID had given me 'time', time I'd not had before as I was so busy. Time to enjoy the beauty around me. Spending my time in this way filled the gap I desperately wanted to fill. That feeling of 'doing' once more.

Out on long walks through the fields I would get lost. I'd often get disorientated but I knew I'd see someone who would point me back to the village. That safety of my neighbourhood enabling me to venture out of my comfort zone. My comfort zone is knowing where everything is yet here I was venturing into uncharted territory. It was the knowledge that the people in my neighbourhood are friendly, nice people. I didn't feel threatened or unsafe in any way. So that knowledge allowed my comfort zone to expand. I could have been fearful of being on my own in the middle of nowhere, but for some reason, I wasn't. I loved finding these new treasures.

I started walking around the village with my camera, taking photos. Then I realised the village had a Facebook page, so I'd post them every day to help others who couldn't leave their homes. Because people recognised my camera, they recognised me and soon I became known as the 'camera lady'. As seeds were sown about my dementia, people gradually began to ask me questions, ask me if there was anything they could do to help.

So maybe the title of this piece should be 'Our Neighbourhood, Our Future' – but maybe that will create its own postcode lottery of occurrence as there will always be those who don't see it as a shared responsibility. So, as someone living alone with dementia, there's nothing more comforting than being surrounded by a neighbourhood that cares, that physically shows it cares. The random acts of kindness left on my doorstep, from biscuits to vegetables from someone's allotment; to simple conversations in the street as people have realised that a person with dementia needn't be someone to be feared or avoided.

My neighbourhood got to know me first as the 'camera lady', then discovered I had dementia. We all had talents before a diagnosis of dementia, we don't suddenly lose those talents overnight when diagnosed. I believe COVID has given us a special time to appreciate what's around us, in the form of people and places. We've all had the time to assess what's important to us and for once, how we can help others close by. So, during COVID, I've given as well as accepted help from my neighbourhood. After all, that's what living in a community is all about.

7

Enabling the neighbourhood: a case for rethinking dementia-friendly communities

Richard Ward, Kirstein Rummery, Elzana Odzakovic, Kainde Manji, Agneta Kullberg, John Keady, Andrew Clark and Sarah Campbell

Introduction

Neighbourhoods have been integral to the rapid changes occurring within dementia care in recent years, although have not always been acknowledged as such. Dementia, like aged and mental health care before it has been absorbed into a project of deinstitutionalisation occurring within healthcare systems across much of the affluent west (Anttonen and Karsio, 2016). In the UK, deinstitutionalising dementia has involved large-scale reductions to hospital beds available to people with dementia and reduced duration of stay (Alzheimer's Society, 2009). In basic terms, it has meant the relocation of care and support from one type of material and social setting to another, and as such marks a changing geography of care. In many parts of Europe, this 're-placing' of dementia care has not stalled at the shift to community-based support. The ongoing retrenchment of public services driven by a policy of fiscal consolidation (that is austerity) has led to widespread closures of traditional council-led day care services (Needham, 2014) alongside tightening of eligibility criteria for admission to care homes and for Continuing Health Care (RCN, 2012), resulting in significant reductions in collective forms of community-based provision. People with dementia are increasingly less likely to be clustered in designated care settings while segregated from the wider community. Instead, policy intentions have shifted to supporting people to age in place through a focus on Personalisation (DoH, 2019; Malbon et al, 2019; Manthorpe and Samsi, 2016). However, as with aged care before it, concerns have been raised over the extent of an existing neighbourhood infrastructure to adequately respond to such changes in dementia care (for example, Miranda-Castillo et al, 2010). The potential danger is that people living with the condition may become, in Rowles' (1978) terms, 'prisoners of space'; facing the prospect of social isolation and domestic confinement as their lifeworld constricts (Alzheimer's Society, 2013; Moyle at el, 2011).

The advent of the 'dementia-friendly community' (DFC), following in the wake of the age-friendly cities movement (WHO, 2007), might be read as a vehicle for policy to address these concerns. Interestingly in the UK, the approach differs between countries. In Scotland, dementia is a devolved matter, with the Holyrood government setting policy which acknowledges the importance of DFCs through the National Dementia Strategy (Scottish Government, 2017). To date, existing development has been led by the Life Changes Trust, a time-limited third sector organisation whose definition of a 'dementia friendly community' incorporates communities of place and interest and has employed a grassroots approach to funding initiatives designed by community groups and evaluated against a set of user-defined outcomes (LCT, 2017). By contrast, central government at Westminster has set out a more standardised 'top-down' approach to community development using a model of accreditation applicable to communities of widely differing scale: 'cities, towns and villages' (DoH, 2012, p 13). Designated DFC 'stakeholders' have been furnished with a Code of Practice (BSI, 2015) including eight suggested 'areas for action' and a predetermined set of criteria to qualify for 'dementia-friendly' recognition. A dementia-friendly community is defined as

> [a] geographic area where people with dementia are understood, respected and supported, and confident they can contribute to community life. In a dementia- friendly community people are aware of and understand dementia, and people with dementia feel included and involved, and have choice and control over their day-to-day lives [p 2] … The stakeholder group should determine its own geographic boundaries and investigate if nearby cities, towns or villages are already working towards the process of becoming dementia-friendly to coordinate possible efforts [BSI, 2015, p 9].

But what does a framework like this tell us about the process of creating inclusive neighbourhoods? And how is 'place' or indeed 'neighbourhood' understood in the dementia-friendly agenda? Here, stakeholders are encouraged to adopt a cartographic (that is map-like) lens, deciding on the scale of their undertaking and drawing boundaries accordingly. The guidance presents place as a bounded container for social action that can be worked on to achieve a set of predictable outcomes. It is assumed that such changes, when made, will have a knowable and commonly experienced impact on the lives of people with dementia. The accompanying model of recognition suggests an achievable dementia-friendly threshold whereby, once attained, lasting changes will be maintained over time.

In this chapter we strike a note of scepticism towards the current dementia-friendly policy agenda and suggest an alternative conceptualising of the 'enabling neighbourhood' (building on Chapter 2 of this volume and Clark et al, 2020). Based on findings from the 'Neighbourhoods: our people, our places' (N:OPOP) project, we argue for a relational (that is, comprised of interconnections of people, places and things) and performative (that is, enacted or comprised of social practices) understanding informed by work in the related field of mental health by commentators such as Pols (2016) and Duff (2011, 2012, 2016). Our concern lies with the gap between 'fixed' representational (that is cartographic) approaches to place that currently drive policy making, and the realities of people's lived experience (Ward et al, 2018). As such, we focus in this chapter on everyday neighbourhood living for people with dementia and their care partners, paying attention to how people participate in the places where they live, and the difference they make to those places as a result. Our argument rests upon a shift in focus from places to practices; thinking of neighbourhood as some*thing* we do as much as some*where* we inhabit. We argue this approach could help in reframing the DFC agenda by placing greater emphasis on the experience and practices of people with dementia rather than the fabric of the neighbourhood.

From 'dementia friendly communities' to 'enabling neighbourhoods'

People with dementia are one of the more recent groups subject to deinstitutionalisation, a process that gained traction in the UK in the early 1990s with the introduction of the National Health Service and Community Care Act (1990) and mirrored across many parts of Europe and North America. Reflecting on the trajectory of mental health services in the Netherlands, Pols (2016) argues that deinstitutionalisation is more usefully understood as a form of 're-localisation' that fundamentally alters neighbourhood dynamics. Pols points to evidence of social isolation, segregation and homelessness in the wake of the deinstitutionalisation of mental health care as indicators of the failure of policy to anticipate the changing meaning and nature of neighbourhood-based relationships. Instead of a narrowly conceived ambition to support people with mental illness to live independently in the community, Pols argues that attention should be turned to 'how people become engaged with others and with their material environment and to the [new] forms of sociality to which this may lead' (p 183). From this perspective, the challenge lies in finding new ways for people to live together, negotiating differences between them and establishing new norms 'rather than importing the old ones – or being oppressed by them – from the "outside"' (p 183).

Pols' (2016) concern lies particularly with analysing how people living with mental illness engage with their social and material environment in ways that lead to new and enabling forms of neighbourhood. This line of thinking resonates with recent arguments for recognising the importance of social health for people with dementia. Vernooij-Dassen and Jeon (2016) (see also Vernooij-Dassen et al, 2018) argue that recent challenges to more traditional definitions of health can be applied to people living with dementia who employ their 'remaining capacities' to engage with resources in their social and physical environment to buffer social health and through this fulfil their potential and obligations, maintaining a degree of independence. They note that '[s]ocial health goes beyond pathology and relates to normalcy and positiveness, and to wider society including its norms dealing with mental illnesses' (p 702). This argument points to an understanding of health as residing in a person's relationship with place.

In his work on recovery from mental illness, Duff (2011, 2012, 2016) takes this argument one step further, proposing that capacities themselves do not pre-exist a person's relationship to place but are created as people engage with the social, material and affective resources of their neighbourhood. Duff is interested in how neighbourhoods can become 'enabling places', through understanding the mechanisms by which the capacity for well-being and recovery might evolve. His argument rests on the idea that capacities emerge from the way a person engages with place, rather than seeing a particular setting as necessarily having pre-existing enabling properties. Hence 'enabling places cannot always be identified in advance, and a place that is enabling for one individual may not be enabling for another' (2012, p 1394). From this perspective, it is what we do as much as where we go that shapes the enabling potential of place. This way of understanding enabling neighbourhoods provides a useful standpoint from which to consider the place-related practices of the people living with dementia who participated in the N:OPOP study.

Project overview

The N:OPOP project was a five-year international study (2014–19) that formed an integral part of a wider research programme 'Neighbourhoods and Dementia: a mixed methods study' (Keady et al, 2014). The main aim of N:OPOP was to investigate how neighbourhoods and local communities can support people living with dementia to remain socially and physically active. The project extended over three fieldsites: Greater Manchester in northern England; the Central Belt of Scotland; and the county of Östergötland in the south of Sweden. In this chapter we focus particularly upon data and findings from the UK fieldsites.

Research design

We used a mix of qualitative data collection methods aimed at enabling the active participation and, where possible, leadership of people with dementia. Project design combined walking interviews (which we discuss further in Odzakovic et al, 2020) and social network mapping (which we discuss in Campbell et al, 2019), and in the UK fieldsites we included home tours, which drew upon Pink's (2009) 'walking with video' method. Where possible the social network and walking interviews were repeated after a period of 8–12 months (mainly in the UK fieldsites). In total, we conducted 304 in-depth interviews over a period of two years. Overall, the project design was guided by a participatory ethos that placed the experience and perspectives of people with dementia centre stage (Swarbrick et al, 2019).

Recruitment and data collection

We sought to involve people supported by a co-resident carer as well as those who lived alone. We also recruited a number of carers whose partners had been admitted to long-stay care. In total, 127 participants were selected to participate across the three fieldsites and of those 67 were participants with a diagnosis of dementia and 60 were carers. The age range of participants was 57–88 years. The majority of UK participants (72 per cent) took part in two rounds of interviewing. Some participants were managing at home without formal support while others had regular visits from different dementia practitioners, including home care services.

Findings

We identified four areas of place-related practices that were linked to the experience of living with dementia and engaging with the neighbourhood.

1. keeping safe: constructions of place and risk in negotiations between people with dementia, their care partners and practitioners;
2. self-care and the comfort of place: seeking out and engaging with places that support efforts to manage life with dementia, including creative and playful approaches to place;
3. holding on to the familiar: the differing ways of reaching out and maintaining connections to people and places as dementia progresses;
4. influencing change: using visibility as 'a person with dementia' to develop enabling neighbourhoods.

Keeping safe

Many of the participants we spoke to revealed their day-to-day movements were the outcome of rolling negotiations with care partners and sometimes practitioners. Hence, decisions about a person's use of their neighbourhood took place in the home, often revealing tensions in the way risk was attached to place in the context of living with dementia. While many care partners and practitioners approached dementia as inherently risky, people with dementia were more likely to view risk as situated and contained. Many had introduced a series of 'place-hacks' to find ways around a particular barrier or threat to safety; for instance, Dennis revealed that he had plotted six different countryside walks from his home that avoided the need to cross a main road. Emphasis was also placed on the need to weigh risk against the benefits of independent movement, as Ruth, who lived alone, explained with regard to the busy road outside her home: "My [support worker] has almost banned me from crossing. I have not to cross the road on my own, I've always to be escorted ... but [friend with dementia] said to me 'you just have to go for a punt Ruth', you know."

Fear of risk was an affective barrier to independent movement in itself, often the vicarious fears of a care partner had to be considered; for instance, Suzanne's concerns about getting lost while jogging focused more on the prospect of her partner limiting future outings than the actual consequences of losing her way. Having lived with dementia for many years, George often played informal mentor to those newly diagnosed and he shared how he sought to alter their feelings about risk in order to embolden people to leave the home:

> 'I said "You've got to 'do a George'," you know, if you get lost say "Great," just enjoy it, there's a nice restaurant or a nice pub, right, "I'll go there and have some lunch." And you always take your card with you: (which says) "I have a diagnosis." Take a tenner with you, or something, enough to get a taxi back or whatever enough to get a meal, a paper, just sit on your bum and read that.'

George's advice centres on the unpredictable nature of place, ultimately the unknowable near-future relationship of people to place, that can prove inhibiting, even destabilising, when living with dementia. Participants described how a 'fog' could descend that led familiar places to become suddenly unfamiliar. In response, a number of participants had developed almost ritualistic preparatory routines before venturing from home, as Judy noted:

> 'Now, I'm going to take my phone with me in case I get into problems. I haven't put my hearing aids in yet today. That could be helpful while I'm out and about. Right, hearing aids in then, handkerchief, yes, tablets. I'm just going to take these out with me, because if my heart does something spectacular, that can be helpful. I'll need a key. I might take this coat because it's thick, if it's cold.'

Such preparations involved an assemblage of objects and practices that buffered people's confidence, a means to contain the anxieties associated with the inherent uncertainty of the near-future neighbourhood.

Self-care and the comfort of place

Neighbourhoods became enabling places through the way people layered different types of place-based encounter to support well-being and cope with the challenges of living with the condition. Green, open and natural spaces held particular attractions. Open spaces enabled people to take their time, find a pace that suited them but also offered a multi-sensory experience that shaped their mood and sense of well-being as Suzanne indicated during our walk with her through a nearby valley: "It's very, very special to me. I just love it because you can hear the ... it's always gorgeous whatever season or whatever the weather and it's just special really, with the stream and the noise that makes and the birdsong." Important as such moments of time-out could be to people's efforts to cope with life with dementia, it was the opportunity to move from place to place, and the cumulative nature of different kinds of place encounter that helped to build a person's capacity to connect with their neighbourhood. Later, in the same interview, Suzanne recalled an experience of travelling to a local shopping centre and the mix of joy and pride she felt in doing so independently:

'I was on my own and there was nobody telling me what to do and I could just walk into a shop ... I wandered around the precinct and had a coffee, sat at a table on my own, oh, it was incredible, it was really, really good and it just felt, you know, dementia – what dementia?'

This shows how movement between sometimes contrasting environments helps to build well-being, a sense of autonomy and comfort with place.

We learned from participants how particular settings could animate their imagination and the value this held not only for a connection to the neighbourhood, but also in cementing interpersonal and sometimes intergenerational relations. For instance, Suzanne went on to reveal how a walk in the countryside could provide the platform for storytelling with her grandchildren:

'There's this tree, its name is the knock-knock tree, because somebody had painted a white door and put a tiny little knocker on it. So, you knock on the door to see if the fairies are in ... and the seven-year-old granddaughter loves going on adventures, and so as soon as we're in the valley she'll say "Where are we today Granny?" And I have to think and we have all sorts of adventures.'

Brendan, who had a keen interest in local history revealed his passion for metal detecting: "Once I find something and I'm not quite sure what it is I'll do research as far as I can and find out." During the home tour interview, he showed us his extensive collection of objects dug up from local walks, many of which had stories attached about their use or function that deepened his knowledge of the area but also fuelled his imagining of past events. The physical act of digging and the material artefacts he collected brought him into direct relation with his local area and its past.

Shopping was another example where material, social and affective resources coalesced with a degree of playfulness to enable people's engagement with their neighbourhood. George was one of a number of participants who took us on a trip to the shops as part of his walking interview: "It's therapy, it really is, it's total therapy you know. I used to like it when my children were younger and we'd go into a lot of these shops and they'd get dressed up in all sorts of stuff ..." Later, as we visited one of his favourite clothes shops, he spent time trying on different jackets until he found one he particularly liked: "I think that's terrific, isn't it? Yeah?" (Interviewer: "Are you going for it?") "I think I've got to." Handling goods and merchandise, trying on clothes, browsing through books or picturing items in their home all involved a playful, multi-sensory, haptic and often social encounter that enabled people living with dementia to participate in their neighbourhood through consumption.

Holding on to the familiar

A challenge of living with dementia was the struggle to hold on to the people, places, objects, experiences and feelings that comprised a sense of comfort and familiarity. In certain respects, dementia could lead to a process of de-familiarisation, sometimes suddenly as a fog descends on a person's cognitive functioning, other times gradually as the capacity to reach out to something or someone becomes more difficult over time. Remembering, sometimes tinged with nostalgia, was one way to hold on to place, in a context where the present-neighbourhood may have undergone radical social or material changes. Tom reflected on his childhood growing up in the neighbourhood where he still lived: "I used to play in the street here. You'd to play football in the street, there were nae cars. You'd maybe get run down by a horse and cart or something." For Tom, the remembered neighbourhood inspired positive feelings and a sense of belonging despite his feeling out of step with the rhythms of the present-neighbourhood where the departure of neighbours to work or school made it feel like a "ghost town" through much of the day.

People held on to the familiar through embodied practices. Undertaking the same activities in the same spaces over and over again was a way of embodying a connection to place. Elsewhere, the 'Neighbourhoods' study explored the significance of the daily walks taken by people with dementia in neighbourhoods in Sweden (Odzakovic et al, 2020). The repetitious, routine treading of a favoured route through urban or rural settings was a way of re-familiarising the neighbourhood through physical engagement. For participants with more progressed dementia, the walk to buy a paper or pint of milk at the corner shop was an interlude of independence and an expression of autonomy where much day-to-day movement was increasingly defined and overseen by care partners or helpers.

Technologies of place were another means by which to hold on to the familiar. Yet, despite the potential of technology to keep people safe and assist with ageing in place, we found only a minority of participants making regular use of assistive or digital technology. New technology was often introduced by care partners, or practitioners, but sometimes met with an ambivalent response from the person with dementia. Speaking of the introduction of a GPS 'tracker' Sandra said: "At first it was quite demoralising, it's not quite the word but it's the only word I can think of, to think that you've always got to have something like that." Murray's wife Gayle had introduced both GPS tracking and a digital camera in the home to allow her to check on his welfare while she was at work. During interview Murray commented: "She stalks me."

Interviewer:	Is that how you feel about the tracker, Murray?
Gayle:	Do you think I'm stalking you?
Murray:	Aye.
Gayle:	I feel as if I've taken control away from him. So as much as it is at all possible, we'll leave as much control to him and discuss things we can't.

Exchanges like this reveal it is not always straightforward to disentangle resources from barriers or to be sure of the feelings they might generate. The social, material and affective can combine in ambiguous ways that fluctuate over time. The technology intended to help people hold on to the familiar could itself become unfamiliar, as Suzanne revealed of her smartphone: "Every time I open my phone it's … I have to relearn how to do … I'm OK for phoning home but trying to find a number that I'm not familiar with, it takes a long time." In other cases, uncertainty over the purpose or usage of a piece of technology meant its potential to serve as a resource was compromised. Much assistive technology was, at best, an ambivalent resource when it came to keeping safe and holding on to place, partly due to its unfamiliarity but also because of the mixed feelings it generated. This illustrates the broader complexities behind and tensions between familiarity and unfamiliarity in people's relationship to their neighbourhood.

Influencing change

Many people we spoke to cited moments in their day-to-day lives where they struggled in public, often in trying to keep pace in performing certain tasks. Paying at the shop till was a key example of the kind of *pinchpoints* that people faced. Lily described one incident when shopping with a friend:

> 'On one occasion I went in one shop with another lady with exactly the same complaint [dementia] as me ... and we got served and got our change and she was holding her hand out and I'm giving her the change you see ... so the lady behind the counter said 'Is anything wrong?''' She said "Have I short-changed you?" So, we said "No, we've got dementia." Well, she set off laughing and she was laughing at the top of her voice and then the penny suddenly dropped and she said, "Oh my God, you mean it." So, I said "Yes, but it doesn't matter."'

Here, Lily describes disclosing her diagnosis as a way to diffuse an awkward situation. Yet, the laughter of the shop assistant indicates the unexpectedness of someone doing this. Not only is Lily challenging assumptions about the public presence of people with dementia, but she is also drawing attention to normative expectations about the pace and performance of shop till exchanges. By making herself visible as a person with dementia, Lily reveals how embodied and cognitive diversity are routinely overlooked in public spaces. Claire similarly described how she would identify herself as having dementia in order to seize opportunities to influence the inclusivity of public spaces:

> 'I was sat there and the manager of [town] station was there and I start as usual a conversation ... and I mentioned to her that I had dementia and things like that ... I was talking about things like the signing in the stations you know. Sometimes you don't know what is the Ladies and what's the Gents and I said "it's not the first time I've been in the Gents," and it's so important that people feel that they

can come, you know that they can still go into town and things like that.'

Susan shared a comparable zeal for engaging local retailers and outlets in her neighbourhood, revealing how the material, social and sensory aspects of particular places played an important role in creating a welcoming atmosphere:

'There's several shops that I've really got to know the owners and I think that's part of dementia awareness. It's a personal approach. It gets you far more commitment from businesses and people. Well, there's too many to name really but one is a cafe that is very dementia friendly. I mean I'm working on the toilets, and that, but we'll get there, but they are just so dementia friendly, you know and the tables really spread apart and it's an open, light area, carpet that doesn't do your head in. It's just everything that ... you know, I wouldn't hesitate in taking my friends with dementia in there.'

John's efforts to self-build a supportive network within his neighbourhood had reconfigured relations with local retailers in ways that had a lasting impact:

'I went into the local shop. I go in there for a paper. They always say, "How are you John?" I said, "I'm going to tell you that I've been diagnosed with dementia." "Oh God," she says, "that's a shame." "Well," she says, "I'll have a talk to the girls and tell them to look after you." I thought it was awfully nice you know. Some staff left two weeks ago, and yesterday I went in and it was a lassie that had just started, you know, and I said, "Good morning, I want this." She says, "Good morning John, how are you today?" And I thought God, it's carried on, you know. She's told everyone and said "you look after him" you know.'

Many people we spoke to highlighted the value of self-disclosure as a first step in renegotiating relations with friends, neighbours and other local players. For instance, Lily described using humour and highlighted how she allowed family and friends to laugh with her over the mistakes she sometimes made. She shared with us an everyday example of how the effects of her dementia had become woven into the interactions with one friend and neighbour to a point where it was just ordinary:

> 'One day I was doing cooked eggs and one broke in the pan and I thought "oh, I'll have that one and I'll give Nora the next one." So, I cooked the next one and getting it out the pan it went right down the side of the stove and I caught it at the bottom. So, I says, "Do you want the one that's the broken egg, or the one that's slid down the cooker?" So, she just casually said, "Oh I'll have the broken one," you know. And that's how she treats my problem, it's normal ... We do have many a laugh over it, but some of it, sometimes, it's just so ordinary, but so off your trolley, we don't even notice it.'

Episodes like this demonstrate how new forms of sociality are being created by people with dementia managing their condition in the context of everyday relations and interactions in the home and neighbourhood.

Discussion: assembling the neighbourhood

Existing approaches to DFCs tend to dichotomise social space and the built environment by approaching the latter as largely fixed and static (Clark et al, 2020). Meanwhile, the social aspects of the neighbourhood, the resources and capital it offers, are treated independently. In this chapter we have questioned some of the assumptions behind this approach, in particular the notion that settings such as cities, towns or villages can be moulded in ways that lead to predetermined outcomes for groups such as people living with dementia. Instead, we have outlined an alternative understanding of 'enabling neighbourhoods' based on a relational and performative view. Here, we ask how does a person's relationship with their neighbourhood enable their capacity to live well, and what are the implications for the dementia-friendly agenda going forward?

Duff (2011, 2012) argues there are three key types of resource that can build a person's capacity for engaging with their neighbourhood and enhance well-being: social, material and affective. Our findings reveal the interplay between these resources in the place-based practices of people living with dementia and have underlined the importance of attending to the subjective and sometimes ephemeral aspects of the neighbourhood as much as the concrete and visible. In a challenge to biomedical approaches, Duff argues that capacities are themselves relational and highlights the importance of the accumulation of relations with diverse places throughout the neighbourhood. His research into recovery from mental illness found: 'Participants who described a large number of enabling places also reported greater confidence in their recovery. This suggests a possible link between recovery and the number and quality of enabling places that one has access to at any one time' (2012, p 1394). Yet, Duff questions whether places hold intrinsically enabling properties, suggesting instead it is in how people engage, juxtaposing one place with another, that the potential for enablement is realised. As such, a focus on the place-related practices of people living with dementia may prove more helpful than trying to establish a causal link between a particular type of place and any benefit it offers (Conradson, 2005). Secondly, Duff has shown that circulating from place to place builds a person's capacities for engagement and well-being as it allows access to different kinds of resource. This is crucial to how we understand enabling neighbourhoods because it directs our attention to the subjective experience of the person with dementia, as an array of place-based encounters accrue over time. Assembling the different elements of neighbourhood enables day-to-day living and supports a person with dementia to maintain a degree of independence (Vernooij-Dassen et al, 2018).

Drawing upon our findings, we adapt Duff's notion of 'enabling places' to a dementia context in two key respects. First, our research shows that the resources people with dementia engage with often have a slippery and uncertain quality, whether that is a result of the familiar suddenly being rendered unfamiliar or the ambiguous responses elicited by certain forms of assistive technology. It may then be more useful to think in terms of a 'barrier-resource' spectrum to acknowledge the changeable nature of people's relationship with the social, material and affective aspects of their neighbourhood. This could also mark a shift away from fixed and binary notions of deficits/assets that characterise existing approaches to community development, underlining the benefits of attending to the work people do to glean contingent resources from ordinary spaces.

Second, we would add the temporal as a fourth barrier-resource with which we found participants engaging while out and about. This includes the challenge posed by what Amin (2008) describes as the 'placement of time' – where time is built into the environment, formally in road crossings or electric doors, or informally in the unspoken but expected performance of tasks such as paying at the shop till. Yet, we argue, it also refers to the way people seek out places that offer greater autonomy over pacing such as green, open spaces or biding their time in a coffee shop. Amit and Salazar (2020) have argued recently that the rhythms and tempo of place have historically been overlooked in favour of attention to mapping spatial trajectories. As our findings demonstrate, pace itself can prove exclusionary, becoming a source of social division that is built into place and yet is often overlooked in approaches that treat the environment as fixed or static.

From a policy perspective, Pols (2016) argues that any new or emerging presence within a neighbourhood poses a challenge to find new ways of living together, and of redefining existing and exclusionary norms that would otherwise lead to people becoming isolated and segregated. Our research reveals that people living with dementia are catalysts in creating enabling neighbourhoods, initiating change through their public presence. Crucial to this process is the act of becoming visible as a person with dementia, and, through this, challenging the 'natural', unexamined and unthinking social practices that assume certain levels of capacity and performance in public spaces. This points to the potential for *affinities of practice* where parallels can be drawn with the *queering* of space, whereby a queer presence challenges 'ambiently heteronormative conditions' (Bell and Valentine, 1995) or when non-white bodies *invade* spaces of white privilege (Puwar, 2004; Ahmed, 2007). Such encounters challenge and change the everyday politics of place.

There is also a material dimension to this process, as people living with dementia draw attention to their experience of 'mis-fitting' (Garland-Thomson, 2011), where the physical form of the environment undermines a person's *visible anonymity* in public spaces, be it through struggling to find the right toilets at a train station or crossing a road in fast-flowing traffic. Challenging biomedical approaches to vulnerability and risk, Garland-Thomson argues that 'the relational and contingent quality of mis-fitting and fitting, then, places vulnerability in the fit, not in the body' (p 600). This perspective mirrors the way that people with dementia constructed risk in the context of our research: as emplaced and situated. Experiences of mis-fitting thereby draw attention to the norms and interests embedded in the design of the built environment. As Blackman and colleagues (2003) have argued in respect to dementia: 'The geography of towns and cities is often experienced as oppressive for many people not just because their needs for accessibility are neglected, but because ableist values are positively asserted in the socio-spatial patterns created by planners and designers' (p 358).

Conclusion

Thinking more broadly about 'dementia friendly communities', our research poses questions not only about where this agenda is heading, and how best to get there, but also about how we can know what kinds of change to make that might be effective and meaningful. Avoiding the prospect of isolation and segregation requires more than targeted support to individuals, but rather systemic change leading to alternative forms of sociality. Hence, new and emerging ways of *doing neighbourhood* might serve as indicators of progress. We have shown that the potential for such change exists, and in many respects has been spearheaded by people living with dementia, who are staking a claim to their neighbourhood often by making their presence felt. Yet, much can be done to support this enterprise.

From a practice perspective, our research shows that facilitating a dialogue about keeping safe could help in understanding certain affective barriers for those living with the condition and their care partners. This is a question of what helps people to be comfortable with place. Problematising assumptions that equate dementia with risk in professional discourses could also prove fruitful. We need to hear more clearly what people living with dementia are saying about place-related risk and how they tackle it. Our focus here on the *doing of neighbourhood* also demonstrates the value of practitioners supporting people to develop strategies for how they engage with place. For example, preparatory rituals can help a person to face the uncertain and unknowable nature of the near-future neighbourhood in a way that acknowledges the dynamism of place, and at times even its volatility when living with dementia.

For policy, the aim of supporting a person to remain independent in a neighbourhood context may be a flawed ambition to begin with. As our findings demonstrate, what matters is the capacity to make full use of the combined social, material, affective and temporal resources a neighbourhood has to offer. This is far more a question of interdependence with people and places, which rests upon the strength of those relationships, even when the outcome is to enable people to maintain a degree of autonomy and a sense of freedom. A relational understanding of capacity (Duff, 2012), and ultimately of citizenship (Pols, 2016) points to the need for policy making that *joins up* the neighbourhood, supporting a person with dementia to assemble the resources necessary for getting on with life. This means targeting support directly at the interface between people and places, fostering everyday forms of connection, support and collaboration to create new ways of living together. It also signals the potential for more creative and collective ways of funding care and support, rather than relying narrowly on individualised budgets and personalisation. Ultimately, it means judging a neighbourhood according to the many different ways that diverse people with dementia are enabled to do neighbourhood.

References

Ahmed, S. (2007) 'A phenomenology of whiteness', *Feminist Theory*, 8(2): 149–68.

Alzheimer's Society (2009) *Counting the Cost: Caring for People with Dementia on Hospital Wards*, London: Alzheimer's Society.

Alzheimer's Society (2013) *Dementia 2013: The Hidden Voice of Loneliness*, London: Alzheimer's Society.

Amin, A. (2008) 'Collective culture and urban public space', *City*, 12(1): 5–24.

Amit, V. and Salazar, N.B. (2020) 'Why and how does the pacing of mobilities matter?' in Amit, V. and Salazar, N.B. (eds) *Pacing Mobilities: Timing, Intensity, Tempo and Duration of Human Movements*, Oxford: Berghan Books.

Anttonen, A. and Karsio, O. (2016) 'Eldercare Service Redesign in Finland: Deinstitutionalization of Long-Term Care', *Journal of Social Service Research*, 42(2): 151–66.

Bell, D. and Valentine, G. (1995) *Mapping Desire: Geographies of Sexualities*, London: Routledge.

Blackman, T., Mitchell, L., Burton, E., Jenks, M., Parsons, M., Raman, S. and Williams, K. (2003) 'The accessibility of public spaces for people with dementia: A new priority for the "open city"', *Disability and Society*, 18(3): 357–71.

BSI (2015) *PAS 1365:2015, Code of Practice for the Recognition of Dementia-friendly Communities in England*, London: BSI.

Campbell, S., Clark, A., Keady, J., Kullberg, A., Manji, K., Rummery, K. and Ward, R. (2019) 'Participatory social network map making with family carers of people living with dementia', *Methodological Innovations*, January: 1–12, Online Firstview.

Clark, A., Campbell, S., Keady, J., Kullberg, A., Manji, K., Rummery, K. and Ward, R. (2020) 'Neighbourhoods as Relational Places for People Living with Dementia', *Social Science and Medicine*, Online Firstview, Open Access, available from: https://www.sciencedirect.com/science/article/pii/S0277953620301465.

Conradson, D. (2005) 'Landscape, care and the relational self: Therapeutic encounters in rural England', *Health and Place*, 11(4): 337–48.

Department of Health (2012) *Prime Minister's Challenge on Dementia: Delivering Major Improvements in Dementia Care and Research by 2015*, London: DoH.

Department of Health (2019) NHS Long-term Plan, available from: https://www.longtermplan.nhs.uk/wp-content/uploads/2019/01/nhs-long-term-plan-june-2019.pdf [Accessed 12 June 2020].

Duff, C. (2011) 'Networks, resources and agencies: On the character and production of enabling places', *Health and Place*, 17: 149–56.

Duff, C. (2012) 'Exploring the role of "enabling places" in promoting recovery from mental illness: A qualitative test of a relational model', *Health and Place*, 18: 1388–95

Duff, C. (2016) 'Atmospheres of recovery: Assemblages of health', *Environment and Planning A*, 48(1): 58–74.

Garland-Thomson, R. (2011) 'Misfits: A feminist materialist disability concept', *Hypatia*, 26(3): 591–609.

Keady, J. (2014) 'Neighbourhoods and dementia', *Journal of Dementia Care*, 22: 16–17.

Life Changes Trust (2017) *Community and Dementia: Dementia friendly communities in Scotland Report 3*, available from: https://www.lifechangestrust.org.uk/sites/default/files/Dementia%20Friendly%20Communities%20Third%20Report_0.pdf [Accessed 23 July 2020].

Malbon, E., Carey, G. and Meltzer, A. (2019) 'Personalisation schemes in social care: Are they growing social and health inequalities?' *BMC Public Health*, 19: 805.

Manthorpe, G. and Samsi, K. (2016) 'Person-centred dementia care: Current perspectives', *Clinical Interventions in Aging*, 11: 1733–40.

Miranda-Castillo, C., Woods, B., Galboda, K., Oomman, S., Olojugba, C. and Orrell, M. (2010) 'Unmet needs, quality of life and support networks of people with dementia living at home', *Health and Quality of Life Outcomes*, 8: 132

Moyle, W., Kellett, U., Ballantyne, A. and Gracia, N. (2011) 'Dementia and loneliness: An Australian perspective', *Journal of Clinical Nursing*, 20(9–10): 1445–53.

Needham, C. (2014) 'Personalization: From day centres to community hubs?' *Critical Social Policy*, 34(1): 90–108.

Odzakovic, E., Hellström, I., Ward, R. and Kullberg, A. (2020) '"Overjoyed that I can go outside": Using walking interviews to learn about the lived experience and meaning of neighbourhood for people living with dementia', *Dementia*, 19(7): 2199–2219. DOI: 10.1177/1471301218817453.

Pink, S. (2009) *Doing Sensory Ethnography*, 1st edn, London: Sage.

Pols, J. (2016) 'Analyzing social spaces: Relational citizenship for patients leaving mental health care institutions', *Medical Anthropology*, 35(2): 177–92.

Puwar, N. (2004) *Space Invaders: Race, Gender and Bodies out of Place*, Oxford: Berg.

Rowles, G.D. (1978) *Prisoners of Space? Exploring the Geographical Experience of Older People*, Boulder: Westview Press.

Royal College of Nursing (2012) *Persistent Challenges to Providing Quality Care: An RCN Report on the Views and Experiences of Frontline Nursing Staff in Care Homes in England*, London: RCN.

Scottish Government (2017) *Scotland's National Dementia Strategy 2017–2020*, Edinburgh: Scottish Government.

Swarbrick, C., Open Doors, Scottish Dementia Working Group, EDUCATE, Davis, K. and Keady, J. (2019) 'Visioning change: Co-producing a model of involvement and engagement in research (Innovative Practice)', *Dementia*, 18(7–8): 3165–72.

Vernooij-Dassen, M. and Jeon, Y.-H. (2016) 'Social health and dementia: The power of human capabilities', *International Psychogeriatrics*, 28(5): 701–3.

Vernooij-Dassen, M., Moniz-Cook, E. and Jeon, Y. (2018) 'Social health in dementia care: Harnessing an applied research agenda', *International Psychogeriatrics*, 30(6): 775–8.

Ward, R., Clark, A., Campbell, S., Graham, B., Kullberg, A., Manji, K., Rummery, K. and Keady, J. (2018) 'The lived neighbourhood: Understanding how people with dementia engage with their local environment', *International Psychogeriatrics*, 30(6): 867–80.

World Health Organization (2007) *Global Age-friendly cities: A Guide*, available from: https://apps.who.int/iris/bitstream/handle/10665/43755/9789241547307_eng.pdf;jsessionid=12010C9B651BCE8C12F91A6B021C94BD?sequence=1 [Accessed 10 July 2020].

8

A conceptual framework of the person–environment interaction in the neighbourhood among persons living with dementia: a focus on out-of-home mobility

Kishore Seetharaman, Habib Chaudhury and Atiya Mahmood

Introduction

The neighbourhood environment has been identified as being integral to the lives of community-dwelling persons with dementia. A safe, accessible and familiar neighbourhood can provide emotional and practical support and augment participation, empowerment, trust and belonging for people with dementia (Keady et al, 2012). However, there is limited theoretical development and empirical evidence on the relations of people with dementia and neighbourhoods explored from the perspective of people's lived experience. There is a need to (1) better understand the dynamic relationship between people with dementia and neighbourhoods, and (2) integrate the physical and psychosocial dimensions of the neighbourhood environment in people's lives (Keady et al, 2012). A major theme explored in research in this area is the out-of-home mobility of community-dwelling people with dementia (Blackman et al, 2003; Burton and Mitchell, 2006). Mobility is central to the ability to successfully perform daily routines and remain healthy, physically active and socially engaged in the neighbourhood. However, currently, there is no integrative conceptual framework that (1) focuses on the processes of out-of-home mobility of persons living with dementia in the neighbourhood, and (2) bridges these processes with individual well-being and outcomes related to their quality of life. This chapter proposes a conceptual framework that integrates the processes and outcomes, as well as the objective and subjective components of out-of-home mobility of persons living with dementia. The research questions guiding this chapter are:

1. How do person–environment interactions in the context of out-of-home mobility of community-dwelling persons living with dementia influence the processes of agency and belonging?
2. How do the processes of agency and belonging in the context of out-of-home mobility influence the developmental outcomes of autonomy and identity?

The following sections will (1) discuss two key guiding frameworks in environmental gerontology; (2) highlight the key concepts from the literature on out-of-home mobility of people living with dementia; and (3) demonstrate the interrelationships between these concepts in the proposed new framework.

Guiding framework

The two guiding conceptual frameworks are the Integrative Conceptual Framework of Person-Environment Exchange and the Framework of Interplay of Belonging and Agency, Aging Well, and the Environment (Wahl and Oswald, 2010; Wahl et al, 2012; Chaudhury and Oswald, 2019). They are used in this chapter to define agency and belonging as interrelated developmental processes that form a critical part of older adults' experiences of and interaction with the environment. Belonging for older adults is deeply influenced by their experience of the environment, representing their attachment to places, as well as the way they think and feel about place over time (Wahl and Oswald, 2010; Wahl et al, 2012; Chaudhury and Oswald, 2019). Agency is driven by actions that are based on goals or intent. In the context of how people interact with the environment, it is expressed either by (1) giving into environmental demands and constraints, or (2) contending with environmental barriers and facilitators to satisfy certain needs (that is through different adaptive strategies) (Wahl and Oswald, 2010; Wahl et al, 2012; Chaudhury and Oswald, 2019). The processes of agency and belonging interact and result in two key developmental outcomes for older adults: (1) autonomy, through continuing to be independent over time, and (2) identity (Wahl and Oswald, 2010; Wahl et al, 2012). It is suggested that as age increases, belonging increases, while agency is most likely to be challenged (Wahl and Oswald, 2010; Wahl et al, 2012). The transition from agency- to belonging-oriented processes in later life could be explained by the increased desire and motivation, as one grows older, to satisfy emotional needs (for example intimacy, joy, social connection), while on the other hand, physical and cognitive capacities to engage in activities may begin to shift and likely decrease (Wahl et al, 2012). The concepts discussed here contribute to the definition of *ageing well*, that is the maintenance of autonomy, identity and well-being despite experiencing loss of competence through later life development (Wahl et al, 2012). These frameworks focus broadly on older adults and the environment and do not specifically address the experience of mobility in the neighbourhood for people living with dementia. However, the concepts in these frameworks can be adapted to advance our conceptual understanding of person–environment relations in the context of dementia and, more specifically, (1) what motivates people living with dementia to engage in out-of-home mobility; (2) their experience of mobility barriers and facilitators in the neighbourhood environment; and (3) how they achieve meaningful outcomes, for example social connection, meaningful engagement, and feelings of safety and security.

In the following sections, we will draw upon key concepts from the literature on the neighbourhood, environment and dementia, interpret the linkages between these concepts, and adapt the previously mentioned frameworks for the purpose of better understanding out-of-home mobility among people living with dementia.

Literature review

This section will focus on the following key aspects that helped build the proposed mobility framework: (1) personal and neighbourhood-level barriers and facilitators to out-of-home mobility of people living with dementia; (2) the different pathways through which people with dementia exert agency and experience belonging in the context of out-of-home mobility; and (3) how these processes lead to outcomes linked to autonomy and identity.

Barriers to outdoor mobility

Cognitive challenges caused by the condition of dementia, for example altered spatial reasoning (that is difficulty distinguishing between left and right, as well as different shapes and sizes), altered spatial awareness (that is being aware of one's position in relation to objects or people in space), and difficulty with spatial memory, planning and decision making, can cause people to become disoriented and/or lose their way (Blackman et al, 2003). As a result, people living with dementia can become fearful of being outside and respond by reducing their range of mobility (Mitchell et al, 2004). The restriction on one's outdoor movement may also be brought upon by care partners and family members due to fear for their loved one's safety (Brittain et al, 2010; Sandberg et al, 2017). Urban areas with high volumes of multiple visual and auditory stimuli, vehicular traffic (Blackman et al, 2003; Brorsson et al, 2011; Lloyd and Stirling, 2015; Phinney et al, 2016), complex street layouts (Mitchell et al, 2004), and inadequate infrastructure (for example lack of outdoor lighting or accessible toilets) (Blackman et al, 2003, 2007; Brittain et al, 2010) further exacerbate outdoor mobility challenges. The lack of distinctiveness in the neighbourhood environment (for example identical streets with a lack of landmark features) has also been found to compound disorientation (Blackman et al, 2003; Mitchell et al, 2004).

Facilitators to outdoor mobility

Accessible modes of transportation are known to facilitate the outdoor mobility of people living with dementia (Lloyd and Stirling, 2015). There are several facilitators identified in the literature that are meant to address people's wayfinding challenges. Being accompanied (by care partners or pets) and seeking wayfinding assistance from passers-by help people living with dementia find their way while outside their homes (Brorsson et al, 2011; Olsson et al, 2013; Alzheimer Society of British Columbia, 2017). Familiarity with the neighbourhood environment is generally found to facilitate out-of-home mobility (Mitchell et al, 2004; Brittain et al, 2010; Olsson et al, 2013) and elicit people's engagement in outdoor activities (Phinney et al, 2007). The more familiar the neighbourhood environment, the greater one's comfort with seeking and receiving wayfinding assistance (Olsson et al, 2013; Ward et al, 2018). Short, narrow and winding streets with fewer less-complex intersections have been found to facilitate wayfinding (Mitchell et al, 2004). Geographical landmarks and street and building signs are used to navigate the neighbourhood environment and maintain independent out-of-home mobility (Blackman et al, 2003; Mitchell et al, 2004; Sheehan et al, 2006; Van Schaik et al, 2008). The use of GPS devices, mobile applications (Olsson et al, 2013; Phillips et al, 2013; Lindqvist et al, 2018) and specialised navigation devices that offer visual, auditory and haptic directional prompts facilitates navigation in the neighbourhood environment (Fickas et al, 2008; Hagethorn et al, 2008).

It should also be noted that besides the role of barriers and facilitators, individuals' perceptions of the risks and/or benefits involved in outdoor mobility also play a key role in initiating outdoor mobility. For example, if the person believes that despite knowing the way to get to a destination there is still some risk involved, they are likely to prefer not to venture outside, thereby restricting their outdoor mobility (Brittain et al, 2010).

Agency and belonging in the context of out-of-home mobility

Agency

Agency is expressed by people with dementia when they overcome perceived mobility barriers by employing active adaptation strategies. These include:

1. choosing to walk when driving is no longer possible, thereby maintaining their outdoor mobility (McDuff and Phinney, 2015);
2. systematically planning and following outdoor routes and using landmarks and signs as navigation aids (Olsson et al, 2013);
3. making conscious efforts to overcome anxiety of disorientation or losing their way: not panicking, calming down, trying to recall the planned route, using all their senses to reorient themselves, using the phone to call a family member for reassurance and wayfinding support (Brittain et al, 2010; Olsson et al, 2013), and looking for familiar and recognisable elements in the neighbourhood to trace their way back home (Sandberg et al, 2017); and
4. training a pet animal to lead the way back home from familiar outdoor destinations (Olsson et al, 2013).

Persons living with dementia also choose to walk outdoors as it enables them to be alone and refrain from thinking or talking with others, both of which are found to be cognitively demanding (Phinney et al, 2007). People living with early-stage dementia have reported being aware that their outdoor mobility may decrease over time. Some, as a result, take proactive measures to maintain their current levels of outdoor mobility (Brorsson et al, 2011; Olsson et al, 2013), so as to continue going outdoors for as long as possible (Duggan et al, 2008). This is an example of the perceived benefits outweighing the risks in order to sustain one's autonomy and identity through the processes of agency and belonging. As dementia progresses, people are known to cope with the increase in mobility challenges by limiting their outdoor movement to smaller, more familiar areas, where they have a greater sense of control (Brittain et al, 2010; Brorsson et al, 2011). They also practise accommodative strategies to consciously limit outdoor mobility, which may involve completely stopping going outside in order to avoid becoming lost or disoriented (Duggan et al, 2008; Brorsson et al, 2011; Sandberg et al, 2017) or embarrassed in social interactions due to difficulty in following what others say (Phinney et al, 2007). This is an example where the perceived risk outweighs the benefits of going outside, as a result of which one's outdoor mobility becomes limited. Adopting the avoidance of outdoor mobility as a coping strategy is known to be associated with feelings of confinement and being disconnected from social life (Sandberg et al, 2017), which in turn could negatively impact one's sense of well-being.

Belonging

Social connectedness among older adults is felt through the experience of attachment, intimacy, cohesion and mutual care/concern from close and meaningful social relationships with family, friends and neighbours (O'Rourke and Sidani, 2017). Social connectedness is associated with having adequate social support and frequent social contact and interaction, which in turn are linked to a positive self-concept of and beliefs in oneself; this indicates a connection between belonging processes and identity (O'Rourke and Sidani, 2017).

Being outside one's home is known to foster a sense of connectedness and belonging to the neighbourhood environment through positive sensory stimulation and social interaction (Brittain et al, 2010; Olsson et al, 2013; Lloyd and Stirling, 2015). Repeated visits to neighbourhood destinations and engaging (that is ranging from non-interactive observation to active acknowledgement and gestures of recognition) with people who are known to those who live with dementia have been found to foster a sense of familiarity in one's neighbourhood (Olsson et al, 2013; Ward et al, 2018).

Relationship between agency and belonging

Research also suggests that individuals' experience-driven belonging may stem from agentic behaviour to maintain social relations, for example seeing neighbours while outside in the neighbourhood and going to talk to them without waiting to be spoken to (Brittain et al, 2010). This goes to show that agency and belonging are complementary processes that are interrelated. The familiarity that ensues from sustained interaction with the neighbourhood environment over time improves people's confidence to go outdoors (Ward et al, 2018) and the ability to maintain outdoor mobility (Phinney et al, 2007), which further illustrates the reciprocity between belonging and agency processes. Familiarity is also experienced through the physical environment when persons living with dementia associate certain personal meanings with places in the neighbourhood, which in turn render those places with landmark-like qualities, and which upon subsequent visits promote recognition and a sense of belonging (Ward et al, 2018). Research also suggests that walking regularly in the neighbourhood as a group with other people living with dementia fosters social belonging. This is achieved through social interactions among the group, the expression of mutual recognition between the group and local residents or neighbours who also happen to be outside at the time of the walk, and raising dementia awareness in local restaurants and cafes (Phinney et al, 2016). These processes would likely have a positive influence on their attachment to the neighbourhood environment. Out-of-home mobility has been shown to foster opportunities for active citizenship among people living with dementia. Some have reported that being out and about is intentional and enables them to practise active citizenship by making subtle yet meaningful contributions in the community, for example advocating for the implementation of dementia-friendly measures in local stores, cafes and restaurants (Ward et al, 2018) and subverting stereotypes and perceptions of what it means to have dementia (Phinney et al, 2016). This, in turn, has been found to augment people's familiarity with the environment, thereby generating a sense of belonging.

Findings and suggestions made in the literature on ageing (not focused on dementia per se) may be useful to further explain the interrelated nature of agency and belonging processes. The guiding frameworks on aging and environment (Wahl and Oswald, 2010; Wahl et al, 2012; Chaudhury and Oswald, 2019), introduced earlier, suggest that as older adults' competence (that is physiological and psychological capacities to function, carry out tasks, and fulfil activity and participation) decreases over time, agency-related processes become less prominent, while processes of belonging gain prominence. This assumption may be extended to the case of progressive decline of the cognitive capacity of people living with dementia. That is to suggest that the progression of dementia results in a greater focus on processes of belonging than agency. The literature on environmental gerontology also suggests that as older adults' competence decreases with age, they are more likely to prioritise the practice of accommodative coping strategies (that is mind strategies to lower expectations from the environment and reconcile with its inadequacy) over assimilative coping strategies (that is action strategies that change the environment or how one uses it) (Golant, 2014). Extending this argument to the progression of dementia, it is likely that the increase in severity of symptoms would exacerbate the precursors for the transition from assimilative to accommodative coping strategies. Thus, links may be drawn between the relative prominence of (1) assimilative coping strategies and higher agency in the early stages of dementia, and (2) accommodative strategies and decreased agency in the later stages. These patterns will form an integral part of the proposed conceptual framework that will be introduced later in the chapter.

Linking agency and belonging to autonomy and identity

Link to autonomy

Being independent for as long as possible and 'fighting back against ... dementia' is considered important by individuals (Phinney et al, 2007, p. 389; Brittain et al, 2010). Going regularly to places one can get to independently, as and when needed, and engaging in desired activities are central to individuals' experience of freedom and independence (Duggan et al, 2008; Brorsson et al, 2011; Olsson et al, 2013). Being outside and knowing that they can engage in activities that they used to be able to do prior to their diagnosis helps instil confidence among people living with dementia to continue going outside their homes (Olsson et al, 2013). The practice of agency through being mobile in outdoor environments partly stems from the support of care partners. Examples of this include care partners trusting people living with dementia with responsibilities that involve independent outdoor mobility, which in turn helps foster autonomy and helps reinforce one's sense of self by building their self-confidence (Olsson et al, 2013). This shows that there is a reciprocal relationship between autonomy and identity, both of which are likely also related to personal well-being. Moreover, being free and independent, especially if the person with dementia lives alone, is linked to greater agency, enabling the person to go out whenever and wherever they want (Brittain et al, 2010), indicating a reciprocal relationship between agency and autonomy. Care partners have also reported letting people living with dementia choose the route for an accompanied walk and take the lead in familiar areas to help them practise their wayfinding abilities (Silverman, 2019).

With the progression of dementia, it is found that people are able to go outside to fewer places independently and become largely dependent on their care partners to support the maintenance of out-of-home mobility, which results in a decline in their autonomy (Duggan et al, 2008). Research suggests that people living with dementia feel constrained by care partners' or family members' concerns and anxieties about their outdoor mobility and safety, as a result of which they limit their outdoor mobility and confine themselves to their homes (Brittain et al, 2010). People living with dementia express a tension between negotiating risk involved in outdoor mobility (that is, important to maintain agency and autonomy) and being cognisant of the need to seek and accept assistance as their mobility challenges increase with time and the progression of dementia (Sandberg et al, 2017). As a result, the increase in feelings of dependence and viewing oneself as being vulnerable (Sandberg et al, 2017) indicate a negative impact on both autonomy and identity. Similarly, in some instances, the family caregiver may perceive the mobile phone as a facilitator to their loved one's outdoor mobility as they can check on them and provide reassurance or wayfinding assistance. However, to the person with dementia, the device may deter them from thinking on their feet and finding solutions on their own (for example seeking help from passers-by), thereby curtailing their independence and autonomy.

Link to identity

Feeling a sense of continuity and sustaining a strong sense of self is also considered important by people living with dementia (Phinney et al, 2007). Being outdoors has a lot of meaning for individuals whose identities are closely linked with the neighbourhood or outdoor environment, for example for someone who spent most of their life farming, being outside is an essential part of who they are (Olsson et al, 2013). Research also suggests people living with dementia frequent familiar neighbourhood spaces that trigger long-term memories and promote self-continuity and reinforce identity, for example taking walks around a local school and seeing children going to school serving as a reminder of one's past occupation as a school bus driver (Silverman, 2019). This may be explained by the concept of place identity (Proshansky et al, 1983), which constitutes place-related cognitions stemming from memories, feelings and meanings associated with the past, present and anticipated physical settings of individuals that are central to their psychosocial needs. Given that place identity changes over the life course of the individual (Proshansky et al, 1983), it may be assumed that the place identity of those living with dementia would likely grow stronger in relation to their environmental past (that is long-term memories of certain physical settings) with the progression of dementia. Furthermore, this theory suggests that their sense of belonging and attachment to their physical environment contributes meaning to their life, thereby reinforcing their place identity and thus indicating a link between agency-belonging processes and developmental outcomes (Proshansky et al, 1983). This theory also posits that the recognition of stable and familiar aspects of the physical environment augment their belief in their own continuity; therefore, their place identity lends support to their self-identity (Proshansky et al, 1983, p. 66). It appears likely that the practice of outdoor mobility provides opportunities for people with dementia to have direct experiences of the neighbourhood environment that reinforce their place-related cognition, which in turn enhances their place identity (Proshansky et al, 1983).

People with dementia consider outdoor mobility as a confirmation that they can do things that they used to be able to do before, thereby affirming their agency, which in turn promotes continuity and confirmation of self, and helps reinforce their identity (Olsson et al, 2013). Inability to go outside and restrictions experienced to outdoor mobility have been found to result in a sense of loss and lowered self-confidence (Brittain et al, 2010; Olsson et al, 2013). Previous gerontological research suggests that older adults' agentic behaviour acts not only as a determinant, but also as a product of their social position and identity (Yen et al, 2012). This finding, when extended to the lived experience of people with dementia, suggests a potential bidirectional relationship between the process of agency and their identity.

A conceptual framework related to the neighbourhood mobility of persons living with dementia

Figure 8.1 shows the conceptual framework that is based on the Integrative Conceptual Framework of Person-Environment Exchange (Chaudhury and Oswald, 2019) and the Framework of Interplay of Belonging and Agency, Aging Well, and the Environment (Wahl and Oswald, 2010; Wahl et al, 2012). Additional concepts specific to outdoor mobility of persons living with dementia are also included as additional factors that influence agency and belonging processes. These are the concepts of (1) outdoor mobility barriers and facilitators and (2) perceived benefits and risks to outdoor mobility.

This framework presents two potential pathways that are mapped onto different points in the trajectory of dementia.

Figure 8.1: Conceptual framework of developmental processes and outcomes related to the neighbourhood mobility of persons living with dementia

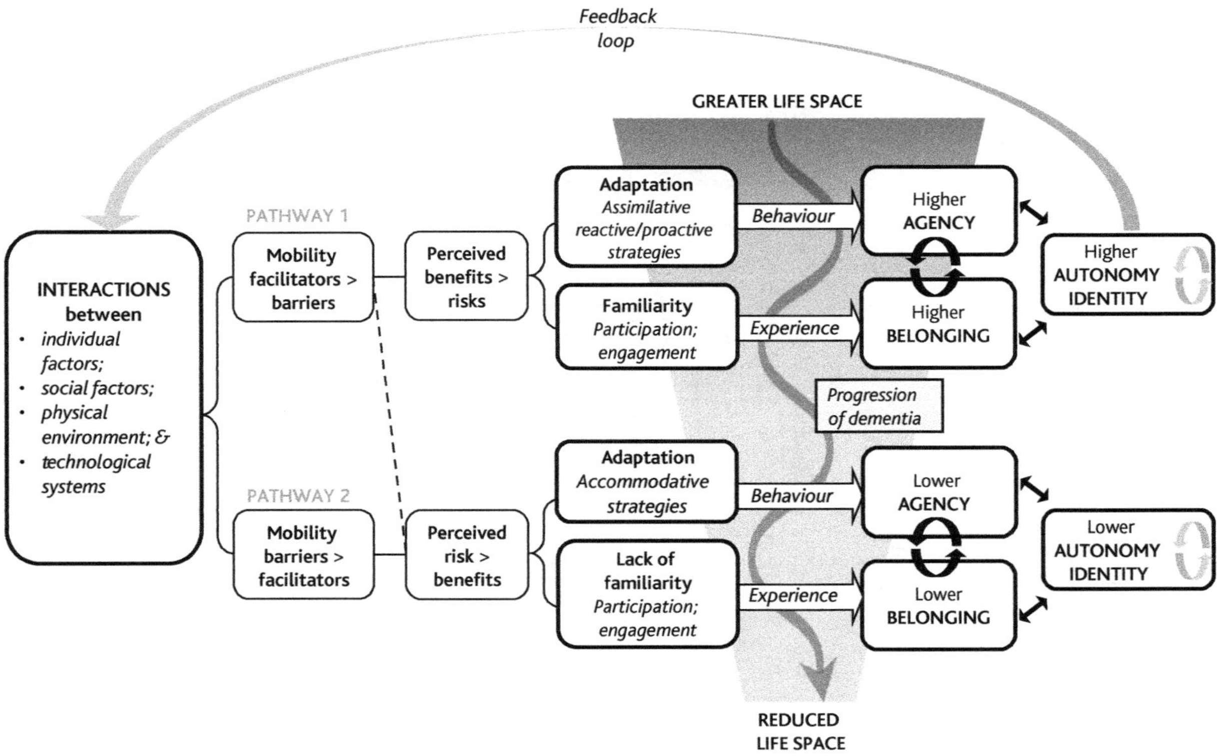

Pathway 1

The first pathway (see Figure 8.1) is one that may illustrate the processes of out-of-home mobility in the early stages of dementia. The pathway emerges from the interactions between the person living with dementia (that is individual factors, such as physical, psychological and cognitive capacity, demographics and background), and different facets of their environment (that is physical, social and technological dimensions). In this scenario, the presence of mobility facilitators is likely to outweigh that of barriers in the environment of the person living with dementia. Owing to the overall supportiveness of the environment and greater competence earlier in the dementia trajectory, people living with dementia in this pathway are able to positively adapt and maintain outdoor mobility by predominantly practising assimilative strategies rather than accommodative strategies. The consistent maintenance of outdoor mobility is also expected to promote people's experience of familiarity through social participation and engagement in the neighbourhood environment. As a result of the combined effect of positive adaptation and experience of familiarity, people living with dementia are (1) able to exert individual agency and control, and (2) develop a sense of belonging. These processes of agency and belonging, in turn, positively contribute to the developmental outcomes of autonomy and identity of the person living with dementia. The enhancement of autonomy and reinforcement of identity through positive agency-belonging processes influences people's ability to interact with the environment to maintain a consistent level of out-of-home mobility. This is represented through the feedback loop in the figure.

The first vignette brings to life the key processes in Pathway 1 through a hypothetical scenario describing the out-of-home mobility experience of a person in the early stages of dementia. This vignette will provide contextual information that helps illustrate the key concepts that are integral to the pathway, so as to make the conceptual framework accessible and easier to understand in relation to everyday experience. The framework has been adapted in Figure 8.2 to help elucidate Paula's outdoor mobility experience in terms of the key concepts. For the purposes of this example, the framework only captures a cross-sectional snapshot of Paula's mobility processes. It is important to note that with more information about the past and present mobility experiences of people, this framework can be adapted to provide a more temporal perspective. However, since the purpose of these vignettes is to understand the key concepts in terms of lived

Figure 8.2: Adaptation of Pathway 1 of conceptual framework for vignette

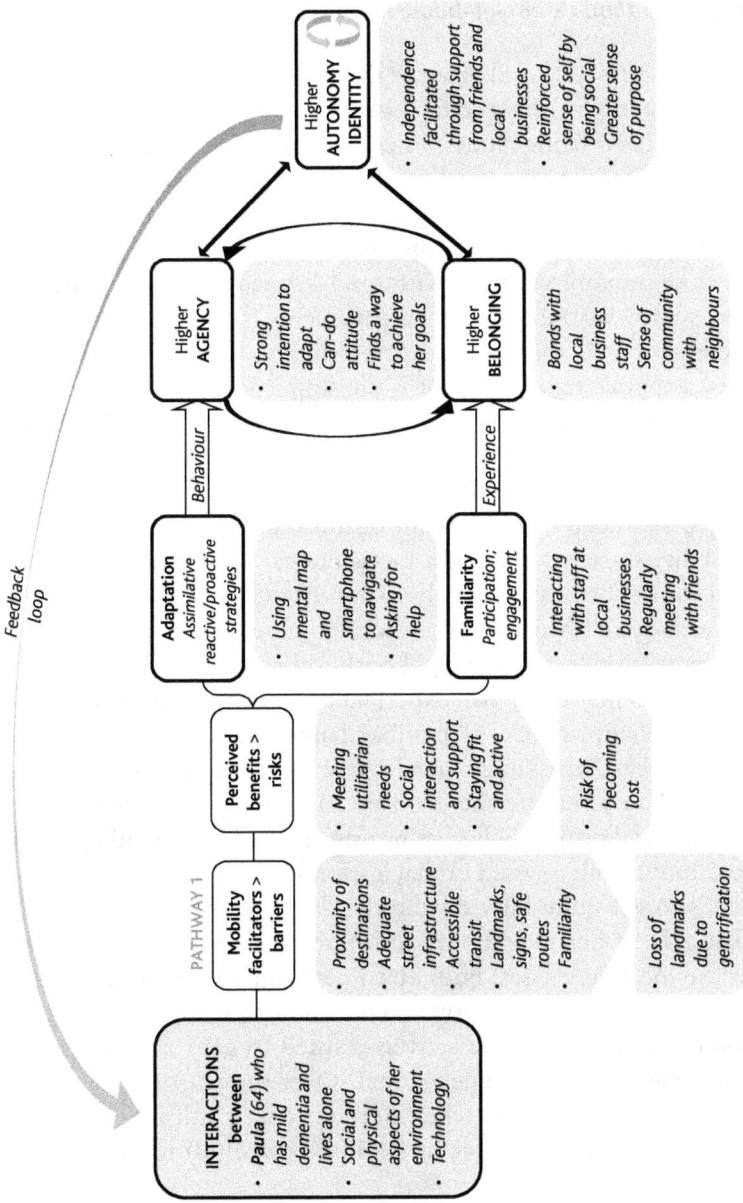

experience, we have provided a simpler representation of the utility of the framework.

Vignette: Paula's out-of-home mobility

Paula is a 64-year-old woman living with mild dementia in a large urban centre in the Pacific Northwest region of North America. She has been living alone in her current home for over 30 years in a medium-density residential neighbourhood with a commercial district at its core. All community destinations (for example grocery store, clinic, pharmacy, bank) that are essential to her everyday life are located in close proximity (that is within a 1 km radius) to her home and are accessible via well-maintained pavements (that is including adequate street infrastructure, such as street lights, benches and signage), as well as public transport (that is the stop is located a block away from her home). Over the course of her residence in this neighbourhood, she has been an avid walker, not only for utilitarian purposes, but also going on long walks in and around her neighbourhood to stay active and keep fit. As a result of this consistent practice of outdoor mobility, she has developed a strong mental map of her neighbourhood and knows how to get safely to and from destinations with the help of well-established neighbourhood landmarks. However, as a result of gentrification in the neighbourhood commercial district and new developments, Paula has experienced occasional disorientation due to the disappearance of familiar landmarks and businesses. These experiences have taught her to rely on her smartphone navigation application to ensure she is on the right track while she goes to the commercial district. This has proven successful in avoiding becoming lost and staying focused on navigation in the commercial area, which tends to get quite busy during the day when she typically frequents that side of her neighbourhood. Furthermore, seeing familiar faces at the local businesses, both customers and staff members, serves as a strong source of orientation and has come in handy a few times when she has had to ask to be actively assisted to get to a destination. She has always been very independent. Over the years she has learned to seek support and help, when needed (that is using her smartphone, seeking help from people at familiar businesses) to continue to live life on her own terms.

Paula is a very social person and quick to form bonds with people that she meets. She has developed friendships with the people who operate the local businesses in her neighbourhood who have become more than just familiar faces and have conversations with her when they see her. Despite living alone, she feels as though she belongs to a bigger family consisting of neighbours in her block, who, for the most part, are all long-term residents of the neighbourhood. They have known each other for a long time and have accepted her reality of living with dementia, showing empathy and support, as needed. Being out and about daily helps her stay connected to them (for example group walking with friends, going to a restaurant with them, having potluck dinners at neighbours' homes) and be a part of communal life. This not only helps her feel cared for, supported and respected, but also gives her a greater sense of purpose and helps her look beyond the limitations posed by dementia and have a more expansive view on the meaning of life and what it has to offer.

Pathway 2

The second pathway (see Figure 8.1) illustrates what may occur further along the progression of dementia, where the person's life space, or the area in which they are active and mobile, is reduced. Reduced life space could be explained by people's restricted outdoor mobility as a result of this pathway. In the second pathway, the presence of mobility barriers outweighs that of facilitators in the person's neighbourhood environment. As a result, the person living with dementia may perceive greater risk than benefits to outdoor mobility. The model indicates (using the dashed line) that despite the presence of mobility facilitators, some people with dementia may follow the second pathway and perceive greater risk than benefit related to outdoor mobility, potentially owing to a lack of awareness of the presence of these facilitators. Due to the lack of supportiveness of the environment and reduced cognitive abilities, persons living with dementia in this pathway are more likely to adopt accommodative strategies (for example limiting/avoiding outdoor mobility) than assimilative strategies and have lower experience of familiarity, social participation, and engagement in the neighbourhood. As a result, people experience lower agency and belonging than people in the first pathway, although it is quite likely that people in this pathway experience a relatively greater sense of belonging than agency, owing to the precedence of emotion-based needs, thoughts, decisions, and actions later in the dementia trajectory and reduced cognitive abilities that compromise people's agentic behaviour in the context of outdoor mobility. Due to the lower agency and belonging experienced, people in this pathway would likely experience negative impacts on their autonomy and identity. However, agency and belonging are shown as complementary processes (that is, indicated through the helical arrow), which suggests that people's relatively stronger sense of belonging than agency may help mitigate the collective negative effect on their sense of autonomy and identity. The person's positive experience of belonging may reinforce their identity to a greater extent than their sense of autonomy due to their reduced experience of agency. However, given that autonomy and identity are interrelated (that is, indicated through the helical arrow), the positive effect on identity may help boost people's sense of autonomy.

The following vignette brings to life the key processes in Pathway 2 through the hypothetical case study of the out-of-home mobility experience of Lee, a person living with moderate dementia. Figure 8.3 shows how the framework has been adapted to help elucidate Lee's outdoor mobility experience in terms of the key concepts.

Vignette: Lee's out-of-home mobility

Lee is an 80-year-old man who has moderate dementia. He lives with his son and his family in a suburban neighbourhood in a big city in the Pacific Northwest region of North America. The move was precipitated by his wife's passing a year ago and the need to be closer to his family for emotional support. His previous home was located in a different neighbourhood in the same city where he lived with his wife for over 50 years. Prior to moving to his son's house, he used to walk regularly with his wife in their previous neighbourhood for a wide range of utilitarian needs, as well as leisure, used public transport regularly and drove to work. Following his diagnosis, Lee stopped driving and limited his movement to familiar places in his previous neighbourhood that made him feel safe and welcome. The move to his son's home has caused a significant reduction in his outdoor mobility, primarily because of his lack of familiarity with the setting. He has tried going on a stroll a few times while being led by his son in and around their house. However, on most of these trips, he has experienced disorientation, causing him to fear going outside. He is unable to distinguish between the houses in the area as they all look the same to him and lack any distinctive features, which further challenges his ability to find his way around. He has a strong desire to be out and about as he did with his wife in their previous neighbourhood. However, he feels that he cannot go out alone and relies on his son's support to walk, which is not always feasible because of his son's busy work schedule. This is the only location for him where he can walk since his son's house does not have a safe and enclosed backyard where

Figure 8.3: Adaptation of Pathway 2 of conceptual framework for vignette

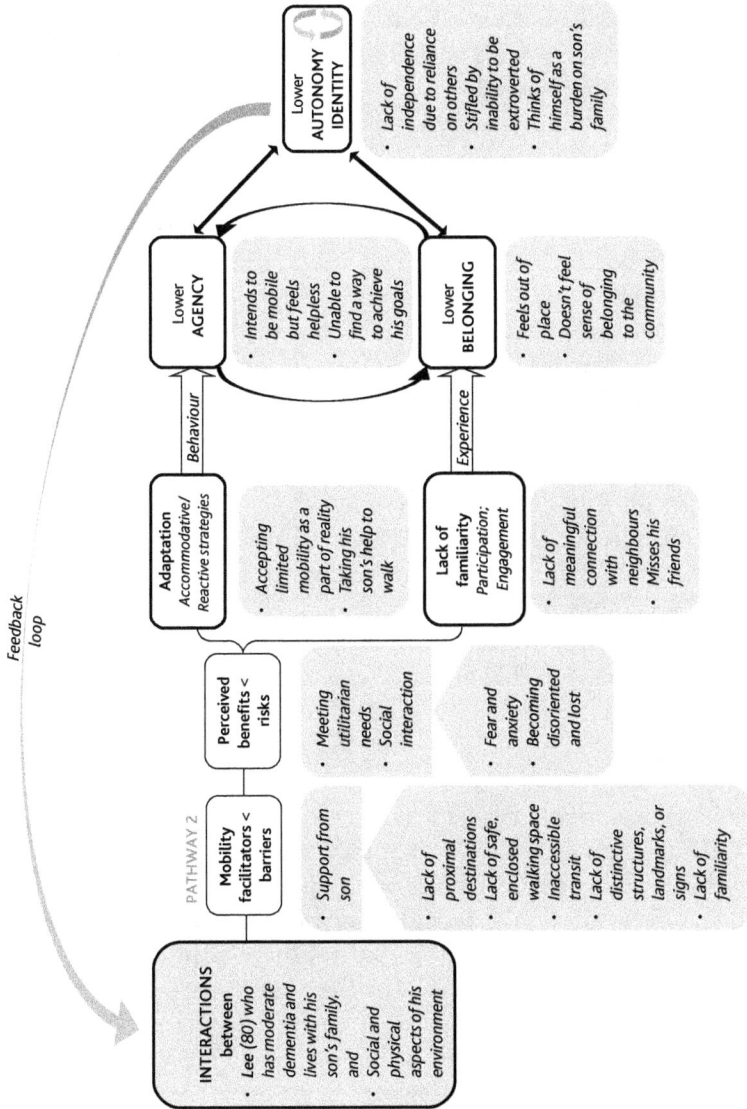

he can walk without running into these issues. Unlike his previous neighbourhood, which had a local corner store close to where he lived, this neighbourhood does not have a local store that he can go to in order to meet his daily needs. The nearest grocery store is nearly 10 km away and accessible only by car, for which he has to depend on his son. He is not fully reconciled with his inability to find a way to enhance his outdoor mobility but is in the process of accepting and making peace with very limited outdoor mobility being a part of his everyday reality. The overreliance on others, especially his son, to meet his mobility-related needs has resulted in an overall loss of independence for Lee, which is further compounded by his feeling of being a burden to his son.

Lee also has a strong desire to make friends in the neighbourhood, especially because he is alone at home during the day when his son's family is away for work or school. He misses his friends and the social interaction that living near them afforded while in his previous residence. But due to his reduced outdoor mobility, that is only when he is able to be accompanied by his son, he has not been able to build meaningful relations with neighbours. Going outside is still a cognitively demanding activity for him and leaves him with few psychological and emotional resources to socialise with people while he is outside. As a result, he feels out of place in the neighbourhood and does not feel as though he belongs to the community. The loss of his social networks has been particularly challenging to deal with for Lee, which stifles his ability to fully and freely be the social and extroverted person that he has always been.

Conclusion

This framework offers a new model to develop a more holistic picture of the complex pathways of interactions involved in maintaining mobility for people living with dementia and how these, in turn, affect autonomy and identity in later life. Previous mobility frameworks in gerontological research have focused mainly on the key determinants of mobility in later life. The present conceptual framework offers unique insight on the processes and outcomes related to outdoor mobility among people living with dementia, by focusing on the interrelationships between (1) mobility facilitators and barriers; (2) perceived risk and benefit; (3) agency and belonging; and (4) autonomy and identity. The framework contextualises these processes and outcomes in the continuum of dementia progression and imminent reduction in life space. This framework advances our theoretical understanding as it bridges the objective and subjective dimensions of interactions between people living with dementia and their environment, thereby not viewing outdoor mobility solely as an outcome or end goal, but as an important dimension in the process of maintaining identity and autonomy. Dementia-friendly community initiatives that are focused on improving the out-of-home mobility of people living with dementia would benefit from this framework. The adoption of this framework of understanding mobility processes of people living with dementia will allow DFC practitioners to have a deeper and more nuanced picture of mobility in terms of agency-belonging processes and developmental outcomes. Thus, by adopting this framework DFC initiatives that are focused on promoting outdoor mobility, such as group walking programmes, and urban design modifications for enhanced physical and cognitive accessibility, would have a wider scope of factors to consider to ensure that the proposed intervention takes into consideration a more holistic view of people's mobility experience. Moreover, the concepts in the framework can serve as key variables to guide the evaluation of the effectiveness of interventions through a person-centred approach, that is by drawing attention not only to the functional aspects of mobility but also to the meanings and values that people associate with being out and about in the neighbourhood. This could mean the development of a survey instrument that is guided by the conceptual framework and helps measure the impact that initiatives to promote mobility have on people's sense of agency and belonging, as well as their overall autonomy and identity. Using such theory-based tools to systematically evaluate current and proposed DFC initiatives to promote outdoor mobility could give us useful information on what practitioners are getting right in terms of successes and outstanding issues and challenges that remain to be addressed.

References

Alzheimer Society of British Columbia (2017) *Disorientation and getting lost: A guide for people living with dementia*, available from: https://alzheimer.ca/en/help-support/im-caring-person-living-dementia/understanding-symptoms/disorientation-losing-ones-way [Accessed 27 April 2021].

Blackman, T., Mitchell, L., Burton, E., Jenks, M., Parsons, M., Raman, S. and Williams, K. (2003) 'The accessibility of public spaces for people with dementia: A new priority for the "open city"', *Disability & Society*, 18(3): 357–71.

Blackman, T., Van Schaik, P. and Martyr, A. (2007) 'Outdoor environments for people with dementia: An exploratory study using virtual reality', *Ageing & Society*, 27(6): 811–25.

Brittain, K., Corner, L., Robinson, L. and Bond, J. (2010) 'Ageing in place and technologies of place: The lived experience of people with dementia in changing social, physical and technological environments', *Sociology of Health & Illness*, 32(2): 272–87.

Brorsson, A., Öhman, A., Lundberg, S. and Nygård, L. (2011) 'Accessibility in public space as perceived by people with Alzheimer's disease', *Dementia*, 10(4): 587–602.

Burton, E. and Mitchell, L. (2006) *Inclusive Urban Design: Streets for Life*, Oxford: Architectural Press.

Chaudhury, H. and Oswald, F. (2019) 'Advancing understanding of person-environment interaction in later life: One step further', *Journal of Aging Studies*, 51: 100821.

Duggan, S., Blackman, T., Martyr, A. and Van Schaik, P. (2008) 'The impact of early dementia on outdoor life: A shrinking world?' *Dementia*, 7(2): 191–204.

Fickas, S., Sohlberg, M. and Hung, P.-F. (2008) 'Route-following assistance for travelers with cognitive impairments: A comparison of four prompt modes', *International Journal of Human-Computer Studies*, 66(12): 876–88, available from: https://doi.org/10.1016/j.ijhcs.2008.07.006 [Accessed 15 April 2021].

Golant, S.M. (2014) 'Residential normalcy and the enriched coping repertoires of successfully aging older adults', *The Gerontologist*, 55(1): 70–82.

Hagethorn, F.N., Kröse, B.J.A., de Greef, P. and Helmer, M.E. (2008) 'Creating design guidelines for a navigational aid for mild demented pedestrians', in Aarts, E., Crowley, J.L., de Ruyter, B., Gerhäuser, H., Pflaum, A., Schmidt, J. and Wichert, R. (eds) *Ambient Intelligence*, Berlin, Heidelberg: Springer, pp 276–89.

Keady, J., Campbell, S., Barnes, H., Ward, R., Li, X., Swarbrick, C., Burrow, S. and Elvish, R. (2012) 'Neighbourhoods and dementia in the health and social care context: A realist review of the literature and implications for UK policy development', *Reviews in Clinical Gerontology*, 22(2): 150–63.

Lindqvist, E., PerssonVasiliou, A., Hwang, A.S., Mihailidis, A., Astelle, A., Sixsmith, A. and Nygard, L. (2018) 'The contrasting role of technology as both supportive and hindering in the everyday lives of people with mild cognitive deficits: A focus group study', *BMC Geriatrics*, 18(1): 185.

Lloyd, B.T. and Stirling, C. (2015) 'The will to mobility: Life-space satisfaction and distress in people with dementia who live alone', *Ageing and Society*, 35(09): 1801–20.

McDuff, J. and Phinney, A. (2015) 'Walking with meaning: Subjective experiences of physical activity in dementia', *Global Qualitative Nursing Research*, 2: 2333393615605116.

Mitchell, L., Burton, E. and Raman, S. (2004) 'Dementia-friendly cities: Designing intelligible neighbourhoods for life', *Journal of Urban Design*, 9(1): 89–101.

Olsson, A., Lampic, C., Skovdahl, K. and Engström, M. (2013) 'Persons with early-stage dementia reflect on being outdoors: A repeated interview study', *Aging & Mental Health*, 17(7): 793–800.

O'Rourke, H.M. and Sidani, S. (2017) 'Definition, determinants, and outcomes of social connectedness for older adults: A scoping review', *Journal of Gerontological Nursing*, 43(7): 43–52.

Phillips, J., Walford, N., Hockey, A., Foreman, N. and Lewis, M. (2013) 'Older people and outdoor environments: Pedestrian anxieties and barriers in the use of familiar and unfamiliar spaces', *Geoforum*, 47: 113–24, available from: https://doi.org/10.1016/j.geoforum.2013.04.002 [Accessed 15 April 2021].

Phinney, A., Chaudhury, H. and O'Connor, D.L. (2007) 'Doing as much as I can do: The meaning of activity for people with dementia', *Aging and Mental Health*, 11(4): 384–93.

Phinney, A., Kelson, E., Baumbusch, J., O'Connor, D. and Purves, B. (2016) 'Walking in the neighbourhood: Performing social citizenship in dementia', *Dementia*, 15(3): 381–94, available from: https://doi.org/10.1177/1471301216638180 [Accessed 15 April 2021].

Proshansky, H.M., Fabian, A.K. and Kaminoff, R. (1983) 'Place-identity: Physical world socialization of the self', *Journal of Environmental Psychology*, 3(1): 57–83.

Sandberg, L., Rosenberg, L., Sandman, P.-O. and Borell, L. (2017) 'Risks in situations that are experienced as unfamiliar and confusing – the perspective of persons with dementia', *Dementia*, 16(4): 471–85.

Sheehan, B., Burton, E. and Mitchell, L. (2006) 'Outdoor wayfinding in dementia', *Dementia*, 5(2): 271–81.

Silverman, M. (2019) ' "We have different routes for different reasons": Exploring the purpose of walks for carers of people with dementia', *Dementia*, 18(2): 630–43, 1471301217699677.

Van Schaik, P., Martyr, A., Blackman, T. and Robinson, J. (2008) 'Involving persons with dementia in the evaluation of outdoor environments', *CyberPsychology & Behavior*, 11(4): 415–24.

Wahl, H.-W., Iwarsson, S. and Oswald, F. (2012) 'Aging well and the environment: Toward an integrative model and research agenda for the future', *The Gerontologist*, 52(3): 306–16, available from: https://doi.org/10.1093/geront/gnr154 [Accessed 15 April 2021].

Wahl, H.-W. and Oswald, F. (2010) 'Environmental perspectives on ageing', in Dannefer, D. and Phillipson, C. (eds) *The SAGE Handbook of Social Gerontology*, SAGE, pp 111–24, available from: https://books.google.ca/books?id=qs6B5isZ6zQC&printsec=frontcover&source=gbs_ge_summary_r&cad=0#v=onepage&q&f=false [Accessed 15 April 2021].

Ward, R., Clark, A., Campbell, S., Graham, B., Kullberg, A., Manji, K., Rummery, K. and Keady, J. (2018) 'The lived neighborhood: Understanding how people with dementia engage with their local environment', *International Psychogeriatrics*, 30(6): 867–80.

Yen, I.H., Shim, J.K., Martinez, A.D. and Barker, J.C. (2012) 'Older people and social connectedness: How place and activities keep people engaged', *Journal of Aging Research*, 2012: 1–10, available from: https://doi.org/10.1155/2012/139523 [Accessed 15 April 2021].

9

We're known as 'the girls' around town: support, isolation and belonging for a lesbian couple living with dementia

Lynda Henderson and Louisa Smith[1]

My partner Veda and I live in Gerringong, a coastal town of approximately 4,000 people, about two hours south of Sydney, Australia. Gerringong is still a farming area, with dairies and vineyards, but is also a tourist destination because of its beaches. We're lesbians: we've never encountered any discrimination down here. We're known as 'the girls' around town. Being well known in such a small town has been particularly important as Veda's dementia symptoms have progressed since her diagnosis of a rare form of Younger Onset Dementia in 2012 at the age of 61.

Even though I've had this house for about 25 years, neither Veda nor I planned to live here in such a full-time way. Veda moved here in 2007 to live with me. Both of us love natural beauty, but also wanted to get to Sydney easily. We liked the idea of a country and a city life. Veda and I have always been travellers. It's something we have in common. We didn't do the usual things that our peers did in their 20s. I went over to France to study and Veda was touring as a member of a rock band.

When I came back from travelling and studying overseas, I lived and worked in the middle of Sydney. It was the '80s and there was a vibrant gay and lesbian culture where I lived, but there was also HIV/AIDs. I worked in the education sector, eventually for the state government, with a particular focus on disability and equity. I was called the 'equity policy queen', one of 'the lesbian mafia'. I applied the Anti-Discrimination Act, the Disability Discrimination Act and the Convention on the Rights of People with Disability to state education policy. I'm a speed reader and cope with struggles by learning as much as I can. It turns out that my professional experience and skill have been particularly useful since Veda's diagnosis.

Veda had a completely different history. She started performing as a musician at the age of 15. By 17 she was leading some Adelaide bands and then toured in Australia before going overseas at 20. In Kuala Lumpur she met and joined a women's band. That was the beginning of what would become the hit band, the *Party Girls*. The *Party Girls* was the only women's band of 20 Australian bands chosen to kick off the first leg of the first world simulcast, Aid for Africa 1985. They had a dedicated fan base.

Before Veda's diagnosis, when I first started living in Gerringong full time in 2004, I started to connect to a group of lesbian women down here. When Veda moved here, I met some of her local old fan club and I was so happy. I thought, "Oh, this is great. You know, now we can have parties and stay at one another's places." We were still going to Sydney but I was also feeling that I had a very nice life down here. But just when these relationships started to take hold, Veda got her diagnosis. She didn't want to tell anyone but started shutting herself off from other people, and she started to get really quite rude. She sort of scratched some friends out of her life and so they walked out of mine as well. That was very hard. I don't think Veda realised how dementia was going to impact her life. I think that she thought she could remain totally independent for a lot longer. She pushed a lot of people away who were offering support.

We used to go to Sydney regularly, stay the night at friends' houses and have long dinners. For quite a while after Veda's diagnosis, our friends in Sydney were a real support to us. Even old work friends of mine would spend time with Veda if I was going to a conference, for example, and she needed a few hours' break. However, most of our friends were still working. I'd been forced to retire early to support Veda, and we had to fit in around our friends' working lifestyles.

It became a lot more difficult to go to Sydney and stay as Veda's speech started to change. She went through some really horrible symptoms at times, which meant that it was getting more difficult for people to relate to her and more difficult for her to relate to them. We stopped going to Sydney a couple of years ago. We've had some invitations to go and stay with new friends living with dementia but because of the impacts of dementia itself, we've not yet managed to do that: we're pretty much 'grounded'.

We used to have a big lunch here, usually on Boxing Day or the day after. People would bring food and drink and we'd have a wonderful party. We did that for years. We had some good friends – gay boys – living nearby. I went to school with one of them when I was 10, so we're like brother and sister. But the thing at our age, in our 60s, people start retiring, moving, moving on to the next phase of their lives. Those good friends have moved away: I miss having the dinners and lunches together. The isolation is really a killer.

We've become much more isolated from friends and family. We've also become symbiotic. It can be a dangerous co-dependency. I have a physical disability myself, for which I also need support, or at least time for rehabilitation and exercise. My health has definitely suffered as a consequence of the time it takes to be a care partner. You end up having to live as a unit, just in order to get everything in place and make life as good as it can be. Years ago one of our friends introduced me to someone by saying, "Oh, this is Lynda. She hasn't got a life. She's a carer." But actually that is true. There are a lot of people who want nothing further to do with me because I haven't put Veda away with the old people in residential aged care. They think I should be getting on with my life.

I wish people had offered something regularly, like, "I'll take Veda out one Saturday a month." People don't stop to think about that. They do with cancer. We did that for people with HIV/AIDS. I remember our community being so supportive of one another during the '80s, caring for one another, visiting. But not for people living with dementia.

Feeling physically and socially isolated, I decided I needed to look for a dementia community. A good friend of mine, who was experienced in aged care, said, "If you want to learn fast get back on Twitter." So in 2014 I did. That's how I've made connections with other people with dementia, care partners, activists and academics.

Being on social media has changed my life. It's changed Veda's life too. It brings the world closer to us, especially now that we can't travel. Veda can watch anything she wants from around the world. She is addicted to documentaries, independent cinema and rock concerts, of course. It was because of the Internet that the dementia community started to reveal itself to me.

In 2014 Veda and I became involved in the Dementia Friendly Kiama project and that project has sustained me. Kiama is another small town just near Gerringong, and it was selected as a pilot for Dementia Australia's Dementia Friendly Community programme. Kiama has a progressive council and it partnered with the University of Wollongong to became a flagship Dementia Friendly programme in Australia. We've had lots of international advocates and activists come and visit us in Kiama to see how dementia-inclusive communities can work.

Members of the Kiama group have become supports for one another. At one point, I wanted to go to Sydney, just overnight for a conference. Between my friends in Sydney, friends down here and members of the Kiama project, everybody volunteered to spend a bit of time with Veda over those two days. Even during COVID-19, we still meet on Monday mornings over Zoom, just to have a social chat.

Being involved in the Kiama project for the last six years has actually made our neighbourhood more understanding of Veda, particularly as her symptoms progress, because we're familiar faces. As part of the project, we've developed our own resources and run community awareness sessions for diverse groups. One of the things that Veda and I do is run around town sticking up posters: we're known as 'the girls with their dementia stuff'. Veda is well known in this neighbourhood. If I'm in town by myself and she's not with me, people say, "Where's your girl?" or "Where's the girl?" or "Where's Veda?" And that's very, very important for her to be known. It's a lot easier in a small country town than it is in the heart of Sydney.

One day Veda disappeared, wearing her red dressing gown. She'd been gone for half an hour, when someone called me and said that there was a picture of Veda on the community Facebook page, saying, "Does anybody know this woman?" She was found. After that, I thought I really need to thank the locals for having looked after her. I put up a post on the Facebook page with a normal picture of Veda and the picture of her in the red dressing gown, with a small paragraph about who she is. There were over 100 comments in just a day or two. It is a beautiful community.

Some years ago Veda said to me, "I suppose if people still remember me, I'd better do something about it." So Veda and I started presenting at conferences. We included her songs and talked about our work in Kiama, and her life in the community. At the LGBTI & Ageing Conference in Melbourne, Veda surprised me and sang a song she'd written for me. I cried. At the end of that, all these old gay boys up the back who would have been in their 70s – they remembered her, of course – were howling and screaming, "Where can we get those songs?" Veda's become a real advocate, honestly answering people's questions to the best of her ability, which has become more and more difficult as time has gone on.

In the last few months, I've started to manage Veda's government funding and care planning myself. That means that instead of using an aged care provider to organise all her support, she and I employ the people we choose by using a broker who supports payments from Veda's care budget. It's hard always having people in your house, but our support people are invaluable. In some ways it's much better organising it ourselves because we can keep our gardener and our cleaner, who are both personal friends now. We joke that Veda's carers are her harem of women. But they are all totally respectful of her background, her sense of humour, her reactions to things, and it's really quite lovely to see these friendships develop. They are all younger than her because she power walks.

When we were trying to choose Veda's new team of support workers, I made sure that she was the one who chose. They went for a walk into town by themselves without me, at their first meeting. It's important for Veda to be able to go out in the community with people who support, respect and understand her. She teaches us all.

Note
[1] Louisa supported the writing of Lynda's story by conducting a two-hour interview with Lynda about her experiences of neighbourhoods, transcribing this interview and then editing it into a narrative. Lynda then reviewed and edited the narrative.

10

Building community capacity for dementia in Canada: new directions in new places

Alison Phinney, Eric Macnaughton and Elaine Wiersma

Introduction

Building Capacity for Meaningful Participation by People Living with Dementia is being undertaken in Canada under the umbrella of the federally funded Dementia Community Investment. This four-year *Building Capacity Project* (2019–23) models a bottom-up cross-sectoral approach to building and connecting community-based activities that provide meaningful opportunities for people with dementia to remain active and socially connected. In this chapter we examine how the project is designed to build practical knowledge from the 'ground up', working closely with people who are most directly affected by the issues (especially those with lived experience of dementia), and taking local context into account using methods of asset-based community development and developmental evaluation. Most importantly, this work is being carried out in two very different places, which is allowing us to both leverage our unique strengths and discover the common principles underlying successful approaches that can then be scaled up more broadly, including nationally. Ultimately, the aim is to create and share new knowledge about how this kind of 'grass roots' approach can lead to sustainable change at individual, community and institutional levels to promote social inclusion, raise awareness and reduce stigma around dementia.

Recognising the importance of place in this project, we begin by describing *where* the work is happening. This allows us to make explicit the significance of local contexts, be they geographic, social, economic, cultural or political, which are intrinsic to how we are developing and evaluating the various activities and programmes. We then lay out the principles and evidence that are guiding the project and go on to explain the project design: its overarching objectives, the approach we are taking to implementation and evaluation, and the project activities themselves, including those that are emerging in response to physical distancing measures being taken in the context of the COVID-19 pandemic.

Health and dementia in a Canadian context

Any conversation about dementia finds itself inevitably in the context of health care. In Canada, our health care system is federally funded and provincially administered. Each province oversees its own health insurance plan, which is accountable under the Canada Health Act to provide medically necessary hospital and physician care services to all eligible Canadians. Community-based continuing care (for example home care, long-term residential care, short-term respite, and day programmes) is organised locally, with a mix of public and private funding. This part of the health care system is not universal. Not everyone has ready access, and in fact, services and resources may vary significantly from one jurisdiction to another, especially where there are different political climates, health care directions and strategic priorities.

Moreover, community-based social services (for example affordable housing, food security, transportation, physical activity, social support), while playing an important role in supporting health and well-being, exist apart from the health care system. Instead, they are offered through municipal and non-profit agencies under various funding models, generally as a poorly coordinated melange with insufficient support and inadequate collaboration across agencies (Kadowaki and Cohen, 2017).

This context is important, because it is continuing care and social services that are the most critical for people living with dementia. As elsewhere in the world, dementia numbers in Canada are growing. By 2038 there will be over a million people with dementia in this country, almost 700,000 of whom will be living at home, either alone or with support of informal caregivers (family and friends). Over a decade ago, the Alzheimer Society of Canada identified an urgent need for an 'integrated system of community supports' (2010, p 54). Today the situation remains much the same – community supports are few and far between, and there is little integration.

This has not been for lack of effort. The provinces have taken various approaches to strategic planning over the last 10 years to address issues around dementia. For example, in 2012, with the support of an advisory panel comprising government representatives and physician advisors, British Columbia issued a Dementia Action Plan focused on health system and service redesign. More recently, Ontario undertook a broad community consultation (including people living with dementia) for their dementia strategy, which was released in 2017 with a budget of 100 million dollars to support implementation over a three-year period.

Canada's national dementia strategy has been slower off the mark. In 2016 the Standing Senate Committee on Social Affairs, Science and Technology issued a series of recommendations for developing dementia-friendly communities based on submissions and testimonies from a range of experts, including four people with lived experience of dementia – an historic event. However, the report itself had little impact, and it took three more years before the government released its first formal strategy in June 2019 (Public Health Agency of Canada, 2019). Improving quality of life for people living with dementia and their caregivers is one of three objectives, with an area of focus being to 'eliminate stigma and promote measures that create supportive and safe dementia-inclusive communities' (p 5). This has provided impetus for significant new federal funding through the Public Health Agency of Canada (PHAC), who are overseeing the Dementia Community Investment. The *Building Capacity Project* was the first of 15 to be funded under a broader call for interventions to increase awareness, reduce stigma and promote well-being for people living with dementia and their caregivers. Since then, several other projects have rolled out across Canada, including a community of practice to support the innovations being developed along the way (https://www. canada.ca/en/public-health/news/2020/01/backgrounder-dementia-community-investment.html).

Considering diverse local contexts: British Columbia and Ontario

A unique strength of the *Building Capacity Project* is the fact that it is taking place in two very distinct regions across Canada. In south-western British Columbia a team from the Centre for Research on Personhood in Dementia (CRPD) at the University of British Columbia has partnered with the Westside Seniors Hub in Vancouver. As described on the group's website, this volunteer organisation 'brings together local seniors and seniors-serving organizations to ... provide an informational "hub" that enhances awareness of local programs and services. It provides leadership in identifying gaps in service delivery and generates community support for seniors' issues' (https://westsideseniorshub.org). Since May 2018, a key issue identified by the group has been how to best help their partner agencies respond to the needs of the growing numbers of people living at home with dementia, and with this new funding from the federal government, they have been able to move forward with greater support.

In north-western Ontario a team from the Centre for Research on Aging and Health (CERAH) at Lakehead University is working with members of the North West Dementia Working Group. This is an advocacy organisation whose mission is to be 'a voice for people living with dementia' across the region (http://www. northwestdementianetwork.ca). Group members include people with dementia and their care partners, and together they focus attention on activities to challenge stigma, promote awareness and education, and advocate for meaningful inclusion. The group has been in existence since 2014 and meets monthly with administrative support and facilitation from CERAH.

With this project, the scope of the funding, and its national mandate, we are able to connect these researchers and community partners, who have been doing similar work but in two very distinct settings, who would otherwise have little opportunity to connect. The geography here cannot be ignored. Travelling between Vancouver or Thunder Bay serves as a reminder that Canada is 'really big' (to borrow a line from a cheeky song by the *Arrogant Worms*). These two cities are 3,000 kilometres apart, which translates to seven hours and two flights, and a three-hour time difference. Being so far apart makes partnering for collaborative work challenging to say the least. Established pockets of expertise have been hard to bring together in any sustainable in-depth way in this vast landscape.

But at the same time, the differences between the two project sites are illustrative of how local context matters. While both Vancouver and Thunder Bay are considered to be 'large population centres' as far as Statistics Canada is concerned (2016), they represent important regional differences. Although the two cities are roughly the same size in terms of physical area, metropolitan Vancouver's population is 2.5 million people, whereas that of Thunder Bay and its surrounding area is much smaller at 121,000. Vancouver, with its population of 630,000 residents (about one third of whom live on the west side), is the largest of several major cities in south-west British Columbia, all of which are located within close proximity, and it is easy to get from one to the other using public transport. It is an economic and cultural centre that has a lot of political influence provincially and nationally. Thunder Bay serves as a hub for a vast region of north-western Ontario, where rural and remote communities are hours away from each other, and some are only accessible by air. It is also more remote from a political standpoint, which makes a difference in how easily community supports can be developed and sustained.

These two cities are also strikingly different in their ethnic and cultural composition. While in both cities so called 'visible minorities' are a growing proportion of the population, in 2016 they comprised only 4 per cent of Thunder Bay's population, whereas in Vancouver they make up the majority at 51 per cent. On the other hand, Thunder Bay and its surrounding area have a larger proportion of Indigenous and French speaking Canadians as compared to Vancouver (Statistics Canada, 2016).

These differences in the social and physical landscape are important. In Canada, specific issues of rurality, minority language status, cultural diversity, and especially Indigenous culture are important factors to be considered given the well-known problems of access experienced in these contexts (see, for example, Herron and Rosenberg, 2017). For this reason, while the project is beginning in these two urban centres, it is designed to extend, supporting implementation into adjoining rural, minority French language, culturally diverse, and Indigenous groups and communities. There are opportunities in Vancouver, for example, to connect with diverse groups within local neighbourhoods to learn how to engage people living with dementia when there are language and cultural differences. And in Thunder Bay researchers and community partners have not only learned to use technology to overcome the challenges of access, but have also taken established models of dementia advocacy 'on the road', renting buses and travelling as a group to small towns many hours away to deliver education and training.

Conceptual and empirical foundations

Overarching principles guiding the *Building Capacity Project* include reducing stigma and creating inclusive community-based initiatives by engaging people with dementia as full partners. As such, this work has been organised around the concept of *social citizenship*, a rights-based perspective in which 'the person with dementia is entitled to experience freedom from discrimination and to have opportunities to grow and participate in life to the fullest extent possible' (Bartlett and O'Connor, 2010, p 37). Such a framework confronts the problem of stigma directly by allowing a more complex and integrated understanding and explanation of social inclusion and well-being in the context of dementia. It includes a focus on social structures and practices identifying the importance of diverse social locations, but also recognises the personhood and agency of people with dementia, the relational context in which they live, and their rights to be treated as full citizens (Bartlett and O'Connor, 2010).

There is a growing body of evidence to support the usefulness of a social citizenship lens for framing the dementia experience in a more positive way (for example Baldwin and Group, 2008; O'Connor and Nedlund, 2016; Birt et al, 2017; Kontos et al, 2017), and that begins to tease out how it might inform practice (Örulv, 2012; Baldwin and Greason, 2016; Clarke and Bailey, 2016; Nordh and Nedlund, 2017; Phinney et al, 2016; Wiersma et al, 2016b). From this work, it appears that community-based programming offers a particularly promising context for supporting social citizenship for people with dementia by creating specialised opportunities that allow for growth and purpose, participation and community, social position, and freedom from discrimination (Cantley and Bowes, 2004; Bartlett and O'Connor, 2010).

There is a small but growing body of literature that suggests that the aspirational concept of social citizenship can be implemented in practice, affirming the importance of socialisation and relationship-building for people with dementia in adult day health programmes (Brataas et al, 2010; Dabelko-Schoeny and King, 2010), leisure group activities (Wiersma and Pedlar, 2008), walking groups (Phinney et al, 2016; Phillips and Evans, 2018), arts initiatives (Dupuis et al, 2016; Clark et al, 2018; Windle et al, 2018; Purveen and Phinney, 2019), and peer support and advocacy groups (Logsdon et al, 2010; Hedman et al, 2014; Quinn et al, 2016; Wiersma et al, 2016b).

However, there is little known about how these kinds of programmes are developed and sustained, nor is it clear to what degree people with dementia are involved in planning and directing these programmes (Fortune and McKeown, 2016). This is important because there is evidence to show that through their interactions with each other in these various programmes, people with dementia are able to construct a stronger sense of self (Hedman et al, 2014), experience greater 'interrelatedness with other people, the community, and society' (Örulv, 2012, p 36) and achieve a sense of 'collective strength' and pride to be making a valuable contribution to society (Clare et al, 2008).

Of course, this research has not been occurring in a vacuum. Seven years ago the World Health Organization and Alzheimer Disease International identified the concept of 'dementia friendly' as a 'promising approach' that rests on a principle of full participation by people with dementia (World Health Organization and Alzheimer Disease International, 2012). Since then several countries around the world have adopted this framework as part of their national dementia strategy (Lin and Lewis, 2015). The UK and Australia are two noteworthy examples of national leadership providing impetus for the development of community-based supports for people with dementia through top-down funding and policy initiatives.

Our work in Canada is drawing to some extent on the *Neighbourhoods and Dementia Study*, which has led by example in the UK, showing how university-based teams can partner with community members, including people with dementia as co-researchers, to develop evidence and methods for understanding how the social and physical environments of local communities are important for people living with dementia, allowing them to stay involved in enjoyable activities, maintaining meaningful relationships, and feeling valued and respected (Harding et al, 2018; Odzakovic et al, 2020; Ward et al, 2018; Campbell et al, 2019; Morbey et al, 2019; Clark et al, 2020; Reilly et al, 2020).

Likewise, our project has drawn inspiration from *Dementia Friendly Kiama* in Australia, which was developed as a community-based participatory action research project to increase community awareness and reduce stigma. Researchers partnered with local city government and other community stakeholders, including an advisory group of people with dementia and their family/friend caregivers. They found that engaging people with dementia as spokespeople and educators was effective in improving attitudes and reducing negative stereotypes across the community (Phillipson et al, 2019). While this initiative showed some degree of positive impact, the team specifically identified a need for 'further research to compare different approaches in different types of locations, and to establish the extent to which *local tailored interventions* are useful to complement efforts at a national level' (pp 12–13, emphasis added).

This kind of 'local tailoring' is seen in initiatives that are more bottom up or grassroots in their orientation (Lin et al, 2014). In many communities there is an abundance of energy and goodwill to be more 'dementia-friendly', and indeed services to support people living with dementia are becoming more common, with initiatives identified in 35 countries around the world (Alzheimer Disease International, 2017). But we have seen that these tend to be isolated efforts; the agencies and individuals involved often do not know about each other, and there is a lack of certainty about how to proceed in further developing these approaches. This is where a community development model can work at the local level to connect organisations and individuals around key guiding principles. But, as noted earlier, there has been relatively little research on these kinds of bottom-up approaches, and where evidence does exist, it is mostly focused on the impact of individual programmes, asking, for example, "how does an arts class improve well-being for people with dementia?" There has been comparatively little work examining the processes by which such programmes can emerge and be supported and sustained, nor is very much known about the participation of people with dementia in these processes.

This is the reason we turned to asset-based community development, with its premise that 'people in communities can organise to drive the development process themselves by identifying and mobilising existing (and often unrecognised) assets, thereby responding to and creating local opportunity' (Mathie and Cunningham, 2003, p 474). Growing capacity for collective action by citizens to produce initiatives that are meaningful and inclusive for people with dementia is now being identified by dementia advocates as the way to move forward, away from a narrow focus on needs towards 'policies and interventions that are truly designed around what people and communities already possess and are capable of doing' (Rahman and Swaffer, 2018, p 132).

Momentia is a prominent example of how an asset-based community development approach has been adopted to build community support for people with dementia in the Pacific Northwest region of the US. It began in Seattle in 2013 as a self-described 'grassroots movement empowering persons with dementia and their loved ones to remain connected and active in their community' (http://www. momentiaseattle.org). Given its geographic proximity (about 200 km south of Vancouver) and the natural alignment between our underlying principles, *Momentia* has been influential in the early conceptualisation and design of the *Building Capacity Project*. It is not a programme per se, but an asset-based approach to community development that works in partnership with local organisations. For example, in Seattle these include the city department of parks and recreation, the Memory and Brain Wellness Centre at the University of Washington, several neighbourhood seniors centres, the Alzheimer Association, and various arts and cultural institutions. It is supported by a Stewardship Team comprising 8–12 community members and organisational representatives who commit to this role for a year at a time. *Momentia* has taken firm root in Seattle, and as a movement is expanding beyond the city as more communities across the state of Washington have accepted the invitation to "help build the movement", starting new dementia-friendly programmes in their own communities that are guided by three key principles: (1) celebrate the strengths of persons living with dementia and include their voices; (2) be open to the public and take place in a community setting;

and (3) involve an opportunity for engagement and empowerment in community (http://www.momentiabellingham.org/momentia-guiding-principles/). While selected programmes under the *Momentia* movement umbrella have been a focus of research (Burnside et al, 2017; Burnside, 2018), the principles-based, asset-based community development (ABCD) model itself has not. Now with the *Building Capacity Project* funded under the Dementia Community Investment in Canada, we have the opportunity not only to take inspiration from this approach, but also to adapt it in different contexts, evaluating the ABCD implementation process and outcomes as they play out over time.

Principles-based project design

We have designed the *Building Capacity Project* according to the principles of developmental evaluation (Patton, 2010), which means we do the work in full partnership with the communities in question, working collaboratively through all stages of the project towards shared goals. This approach is action oriented, focusing on the co-creation of knowledge for the purpose of supporting social change, and specifically allows us to address community-identified issues as they emerge. It is not a methodology in and of itself, but rather a set of principles that democratises the research process, supporting the use of different methods that are being chosen in accordance with the conceptual underpinnings and practical aims of the work as it moves ahead. As the term implies, the approach is particularly suited to interventions in their developmental phases and guiding them in complex community contexts that may shift over time.

The *Building Capacity Project* is addressing three specific aims:

1. *implement an asset-based community development approach* to adapt and create community programmes and services that are meaningful and inclusive for people with dementia;
2. *conduct a developmental evaluation* that will allow us to learn along the way how to best support the growth and integration of programmes and services that are meaningful and inclusive for people with dementia;
3. *disseminate what we learn from this project* to increase community awareness about dementia and to support communities in their sustained efforts to create opportunities for meaningful participation by people with dementia.

Our commitment to social citizenship is meant to ensure that people with dementia are engaged through all aspects of the project, not just brought in as 'service users' or 'program participants'. Thunder Bay is leading the charge in this regard. Here the project is co-led by a steering committee of people living with dementia drawn from the North West [Ontario] Dementia Working Group. As an experienced group of advocates, they have been providing education and awareness-raising activities, and advocating for inclusion around the region, showing through their own actions how to effectively engage the meaningful participation of people living with dementia.

The context is quite different in Vancouver, where the impetus for the project has come from the Westside Seniors Hub, who are bringing their partner agencies together to do more in support of people with dementia who are living in the neighbourhood. But these groups do not yet identify as working *with* people with dementia. Therefore, some of the early activities in Vancouver have involved training to develop skills and confidence, and identifying strategies for reaching out to connect with people with lived experience of dementia.

In a sense, then, we see two different approaches to our community development work – from the 'inside out' and from the 'outside in'. Creating community change often happens in organic grassroots ways, and by having two different models of community change, we have the opportunity to observe how each approach works. In Thunder Bay the initiatives are developed and initiated by people with lived experience who are advocating for inclusion. In Vancouver social change is being driven by community partners who want to be more inclusive of people living with dementia. These two different approaches offer important learning as we move forward with building dementia-inclusive communities.

A social citizenship lens not only foregrounds the individual experiences of a person living with dementia, but also addresses their *social location*, which leads us to explicitly consider matters of diversity. For example, it has been recognised that people with dementia in community leadership and advocacy positions tend to be young (often under 65) and male, which is not at all representative of the larger population of people living with dementia (Alzheimer Disease International, 2015). Throughout the project we are paying close attention to how programmes can be developed to ensure access and participation by people with dementia of different genders and ages, cultures and socio-economic backgrounds. For example, in Vancouver the Westside Seniors Hub is discussing the limitations they face in the fact that as a group they are mostly white English-speaking people, which does not reflect the cultural make-up of their neighbourhood. They are considering how to extend their reach to connect with other cultural groups, including Indigenous people, and families who do not speak English as a first language.

Project activities

Guided by the asset-based community development approach (Mathie and Cunningham, 2003; Green-Harris et al, 2019), the project has begun with an asset mapping exercise in each city, that is, stakeholder interviews and primary research aimed at building broader awareness of and extending connections between existing community resources. This is related not only to existing programmes, but to the broader physical, social and cultural assets of each neighbourhood. This will provide a foundation for activities across the four years of the project, including:

- *community conversations* (for example meetings, focus groups, and panel discussions) to increase knowledge and awareness across the community;
- *workshops and community events to engage people living with dementia* to ensure that they have meaningful involvement in planning, implementation and evaluation activities, and that community members have increased comfort, knowledge and skills to support this kind of involvement;
- *networking and sharing success stories* so communities and individuals will have more opportunity to connect and communicate 'what works', and have increased enthusiasm for innovation;
- *new dementia initiatives* (social and physical activities, arts programmes, volunteer opportunities and so on) that will create expanded opportunities for engagement by people living with dementia and build organisational confidence and commitment to sustain such initiatives through the longer term.

As programmes and services are being adapted and created, evaluation activities will be integrated through the years of the project, employing a range of methods including interviews, focus groups, observation, surveys and mapping activities, document analysis and social network analysis. As a developmental evaluation, the goal is not only to demonstrate robust project outcomes, but also, equally important, to support community organisations to create their own evaluation strategies that are both meaningful and feasible, and inclusive of people living with dementia and that can be sustained after the project is complete.

Dissemination activities will also be integrated through the years of the project. These will include ongoing *grassroots promotional activities* to increase awareness and knowledge among community members, people living with dementia, families, researchers and decision makers; *rapid feedback and evaluation reports* to give those who are developing and implementing new initiatives access to the most recent evaluation feedback so they can make changes 'on the fly'; and *regular project updates* to improve the capacity of the local community to develop more initiatives and to 'spread the word' so other communities will have resources to try similar approaches. At the end of the project a range of knowledge products are expected, including a national forum and final written reports, tool kits and video case studies.

Implementation and evaluation methods

In our effort to determine 'what works', we are using principles-focused evaluation (Patton, 2018), which is seen to be particularly appropriate for implementing community interventions in complex contexts, where both the intervention and the community feature complexity. Complex interventions are ones that feature multiple components that may interact unpredictably, and have outcomes at various levels within the community (that is at the individual, programme, agency, neighbourhood and systems levels). A more traditional approach would seek to build knowledge about 'best practices' and then base any subsequent implementation strategy on ensuring 'fidelity' to the intervention's presumed critical ingredients. However, there is an evolving understanding that 'top-down' approaches such as this are not appropriate; instead, the better way to navigate complex community contexts is to articulate guiding principles (some a priori, some emergent), test whether these are actually being put into practice, and then analyse whether and how the principles are having an impact on the valued outcomes (Hawe, 2015).

A key premise in this kind of evaluation is that engaging community leaders and key stakeholders throughout the research results in more relevant research questions, as well as better-designed interventions, and thus ultimately in greater capacity for sustaining and spreading the knowledge about what works. This aligns also with the underpinnings of social citizenship and our commitment to focus explicitly on the insights and experiences of community members who themselves are living with dementia. Research on dementia often does not take the perspectives of people with dementia into account. For example, though most people with dementia live in the community, 'existing studies may not meaningfully reflect outcome measures of importance for people living at home' (Morbey et al, 2019, p 2). It is increasingly recognised that these different perspectives need to be understood and valued, whether it is through the creation of 'safe spaces' where people with dementia can share their experiences without the 'intrusion' of caregivers (Wiersma et al, 2016b), or by mapping innovative methods (for example arts-based approaches, visual methods, action research, and so on) for engaging people with dementia in health care and research (Phillipson and Hammond, 2018). This project is allowing us to implement these ideas within the project's two different geographic contexts in a way that could be scaled up more broadly in the future.

Early learnings

In the face of the vast physical distance between Vancouver and Thunder Bay, one key early learning point has been the importance of hosting an in-person launch event. In February 2020 the members of the Thunder Bay team came to Vancouver so everyone could meet and orient each other to their local contexts and activities, and learn from others who shared success stories about moving ideas of social citizenship into action (for example representatives from *Momentia* in Seattle). Out of the event has come the realisation that the two sites have different but complementary strengths which offer the potential for valuable mutual learning going forward: Thunder Bay has strong direct involvement and experience with engagement of people with lived experience of dementia, but relatively few ongoing relationships with community agencies. As a smaller city with fewer resources and a more expansive geography, it may simply be more challenging to support meaningful participation in this way. Vancouver, on the other hand, with its rich history of neighbourhood engagement and social activism, has strong relationships with a variety of community partners (community centres, seniors' centres, day programmes, libraries, and so on), but is only starting to include people with lived experience in this work.

The in-person interactions that happened during this two-day event have been essential for grounding our working relationships going forward, which turned out to be even more crucial once the pandemic was declared three weeks later. Since then, building on these relationships, we have hosted a series of cross-site webinars aimed at helping community partners envision how they can adapt their planned activities going forward in the context of the pandemic, and sharing ideas about how the respective strengths of our two sites – one working from the 'outside in' and the other from the 'inside out' – can be merged going forward for the benefit of people living with dementia. Community members in both provinces have been able to share their early successes (for example figuring out the logistics of bringing people into social spaces online) and learn from each other better ways to engage people living with dementia.

At the same time, early experiences in the two sites show some striking differences in how processes are being tailored as we move forward. In Thunder Bay the Northwest Dementia Working Group has been forced to acknowledge that the work they had started in 2019 to connect with rural and remote communities several hours distant from the city has had to stop due to the social distancing measures and travel limitations of COVID-19. For a while they found themselves turning more inward, nurturing relationships among themselves and finding ways to support each other through the pandemic. But it seems that this could be building their capacity for a different kind of engagement as they begin to consider letter-writing and media campaigns directed at their provincial government, advocating for rights for people with dementia.

In Vancouver, on the other hand, there are established not-for-profit community groups who have found ways to maintain and even create new opportunities to engage people with dementia. Building on the relationships forged during our February 2020 launch event, and fostered during the pandemic through online webinars, they are sharing implementation insights (for example how to shift a dementia cafe online), and creating new collaborations, such as a cross-agency partnership to develop opportunities for people to get outside safely. An important insight has been the necessity of taking a 'small wins' approach (Weick, 1984) to effecting change, particularly within the context of required social distancing.

Conclusion

The *Building Capacity Project* offers a window of opportunity in Canada to connect with and build on new initiatives supporting social citizenship in dementia, both *globally* (drawing inspiration from community-engaged innovations in the UK, US and Australia) and *locally* (leveraging people's desire to make a real difference in their own neighbourhoods). We are moving forward on the belief that working from the ground up is a powerful model for enacting sustainable change. Through collective action, and in partnership with people who are living with dementia, our shared goal is that after four years there will be many more people with dementia who are active and participating in self-advocacy, leadership and community life. More importantly, we want there to be greater social capacity for this kind of active participation to grow and flourish, showing through example that dementia does not inevitably result in withdrawal from the world.

This project aims to reduce stigma and increase awareness of what it takes to support the rights of people with dementia to live well and participate as social citizens. This kind of positive social change is not just a matter of spreading good ideas of social citizenship and inclusion, but figuring out how to put these ideas into action in *diverse local contexts*. Through an approach of asset-based community development and an evaluation model focused on shared principles, the *Building Capacity Project* is showing how the unique political, social and physical landscapes of British Columbia and northern Ontario influence how local communities are learning to get things done in a way that works best for them.

Through developmental evaluation, this project has been designed to uncover and embrace the *complexity* that is inherent in such an endeavour. For other communities seeking to do something similar in the future, this should result not in a set of checklists necessarily, but rather in a set of guiding principles, and examples showing different pathways to success. Of course, none of us predicted something as different as a pandemic that would prevent people from physically coming together; community development with everyone at home has been a real test. And yet, it has forced us to think in a more careful and considered way about how the virtual world has become perhaps a kind of *third place* in this project, one where the challenges of geographic distance and mobility have fallen away to some degree and we are seeing pathways towards the development of new approaches to creating practical and meaningful opportunities for people with dementia to remain as active social citizens.

References

Alzheimer's Disease International [ADI] (2015) 'Women and dementia: A global research review', available from: https://www.alz.co.uk/sites/default/files/pdfs/Women-and-Dementia.pdf

Alzheimer's Disease International (2017) *Dementia Friendly Communities: Global Developments*, 2nd edn, London: Alzheimer's Disease International.

Alzheimer Society of Canada (2010) *The Rising Tide: The Impact of Dementia on Canadian Society*, Toronto: Alzheimer Society.

Baldwin, C. and Greason, M. (2016) 'Micro-citizenship, dementia and long-term care', *Dementia*, 15(3): 289–303.

Baldwin, C. and Group, B.D. (2008) 'Narrative(,) citizenship and dementia: The personal and the political', *Journal of Aging Studies*, 22(3): 222–8.

Bartlett, R. and O'Connor, D. (2010) *Broadening the Dementia Debate: Toward Social Citizenship*, Bristol: Policy Press.

Birt, L., Poland, F., Csipke, E. and Charlesworth, G. (2017) 'Shifting dementia discourses from deficit to active citizenship', *Sociology of Health & Illness*, 3(2): 199–211.

Brataas, H., Bjugan, H., Wille, T. and Hellzen, O. (2010) 'Experiences of day care and collaboration among people with mild dementia', *Journal of Clinical Nursing*, 19: 2839–48.

Burnside, L. (2018) *'Just a Moment' Musical Theater for Persons with Dementia and their Care Partners*, 47th Annual Scientific and Educational Meeting, Canadian Association on Gerontology, Vancouver, BC.

Burnside, L.D., Knecht, M.J., Hopley, E.K. and Logsdon, R.G. (2017) 'Here: now –Conceptual model of the impact of an experiential arts program on persons with dementia and their care partners', *Dementia*, 16(1): 29–45.

Campbell, S., Clark, A., Keady, J., Kullberg, A., Manji, K., Rummery, K. and Ward, R. (2019) 'Participatory social network map making with family carers of people living with dementia', *Methodological Innovations*, 12(1): 2059799119844445.

Cantley, C. and Bowes, A. (2004) 'Dementia and social inclusion: The way forward', in Innes, A., Archibold, K. and Murphy, C. (eds) *Dementia and Social Inclusion: Marginalized Groups and Marginalized Areas of Dementia Research, Care and Practice*, London: Jessica Kingsley, pp 255–71.

Clare, L., Rowlands, J.M. and Quin, R. (2008) 'Collective strength: The impact of developing a shared social identity in early-stage dementia', *Dementia*, 7(1): 9–30.

Clark, A.J., Campbell, S., Keady, J., Kullberg, A., Manji, A., Rummery, K. and Ward, R. (2020) 'Neighbourhoods as relational places for people living with dementia', *Social Science and Medicine*, 252: 112927.

Clark, I.N., Tamplin, J.D. and Baker, F.A. (2018) 'Community-dwelling people living with dementia and their family caregivers experience enhanced relationships and feelings of well-being following therapeutic group singing: A qualitative thematic analysis', *Frontiers in Psychology*, Jul 30(9): 1332.

Clarke, C.L. and Bailey, C. (2016) 'Narrative citizenship, resilience and inclusion with dementia: On the inside or on the outside of physical and social places', *Dementia*, 15(3): 434–52.

Dabelko-Schoeny, H. and King, S. (2010) 'In their own words: Participants' perceptions of the impact of adult day services', *Journal of Gerontological Social Work*, 53: 176–92.

Dupuis, S.L., Kontos, P., Mitchell, G., Jonas-Simpson, C. and Gray, J. (2016) 'Re-claiming citizenship through the arts', *Dementia: The International Journal of Social Research and Practice*, 15(3): 358–80.

Fortune, D. and McKeown, J. (2016) 'Sharing the journey: Exploring a social leisure program for persons with dementia and their spouses', *Leisure Sciences*, 38: 373–87.

Green-Harris, G., Coley, S.L., Koscik, R.L., Norris, N.C., Houston, S.L., Sager, M.A., Johnson, S.C. and Edwards, D.F. (2019) 'Addressing disparities in Alzheimer's disease and African-American participation in research: An asset-based community development approach', *Frontiers in Aging Neuroscience*, 11: 125.

Harding, A.J.E., Morbey, H., Ahmed, F., Opdebeeck, C., Wang, Y-Y., Williamson, P., Leroi, I., Challis, D., Davies, L., Reeves, D., Holland, F., Hann, M., Hellström, I., Hydén L-C., Burns, A., Keady, J. and Reilly, S. (2018) 'Developing a core outcome set for people living with dementia at home in their neighbourhoods and communities: Study protocol for use in the evaluation of non-pharmacological community-based health and social care interventions', *Trials*, 19(1): 1–13.

Hawe, P. (2015) 'Lessons from complex interventions to improve health', *Annual Review of Public Health*, 36: 307–23.

Hedman, R., Hellström, I., Ternestedt, B.M., Hansebo, G. and Norberg, A. (2014) 'Social positioning by people with Alzheimer's disease in a support group', *Journal of Aging Studies*, 28: 11–21.

Herron, R.V. and Rosenberg, M.W. (2017) '"Not there yet": Examining community support from the perspective of people with dementia and their partners in care', *Social Science & Medicine*, 173: 81–7.

Kadowaki, L. and Cohen, M. (2017) *Raising the Profile of Community-based Seniors' Services Sector in B.C.: A Review of the Literature*, available from: www.seniorsraisingtheprofile.ca

Kontos, P., Miller, K.L. and Kontos, A.P. (2017) 'Relational citizenship: Supporting embodied selfhood and relationality in dementia care', *Sociology of Health & Illness*, 39(2): 182–98.

Lin, S.Y., Becker, M. and Belza, B. (2014) 'From dementia fearful to dementia friendly: Be a champion in your community', *Journal of Gerontological Nursing*, 40(12): 3–5.

Lin, S.Y. and Lewis, F.M. (2015) 'Dementia friendly, dementia capable, and dementia positive: Concepts to prepare for the future', *The Gerontologist*, 55(2): 237–44.

Logsdon, R.G., Pike, K.C., McCurry, S.M., Hunter, P., Maher, J., Snyder, L. and Teri, L. (2010) 'Early-stage memory loss support groups: Outcomes from a randomized controlled clinical trial', *Journals of Gerontology, Series B: Psychological Sciences and Social Sciences*, 65B: 691–7.

Mathie, A. and Cunningham, G. (2003) 'From clients to citizens: Asset-based community development as a strategy for community-driven development', *Development in Practice*, 13(5): 474–86.

Morbey, H., Harding, A.J.E., Swarbrick, C., Ahmed, F., Elvish, R., Keady, J., Williamson, P.R. and Reilly, S.T. (2019) 'Involving people living with dementia in research: An accessible modified Delphi survey for core outcome set development', *Trials*, 20 (12), available from: https://doi.org/10.1186/s13063-018-3069-6 [Accessed 15 April 2021].

Nordh, J. and Nedlund, A.-C. (2017) 'To coordinate information in practice: Dilemmas and strategies in care management for citizens with dementia', *Journal of Social Service Research*, 43(3): 319–35. DOI: 10.1080/01488376.2016.1217580

O'Connor, D. and Nedlund, A.C. (2016) 'Editorial introduction: Special issue on citizenship and dementia', *Dementia*, 15(3): 285–8.

Odzakovic, E., Hellström, I., Ward, R. and Kullberg, A. (2020) '"Overjoyed that I can go outside": Using walking interviews to learn about the lived experience and meaning of neighbourhood for people living with dementia', *Dementia*, 19(7): 2199–219, 1471301218817453

Örulv, L. (2012) 'Reframing dementia in Swedish self-help group conversations: Constructing citizenship', *International Journal of Self Help and Self Care*, 6(1): 9.

Patton, M.Q. (2010) *Developmental Evaluation: Applying Complexity Concepts to Enhance Innovation and Use*, New York: Guilford Press.

Patton, M.Q. (2018) *Principles-focused Evaluation: The Guide*, New York: Guilford Press.

Phillips, R. and Evans, B. (2018) 'Friendship, curiosity and the city: Dementia friends and memory walks in Liverpool', *Urban Studies*, 55(3): 639–54.

Phillipson, L., Hall, D., Cridland, E., Fleming, R., Brennan-Horley, C., Guggisberg, N., Frost, D. and Hasan, H. (2019) 'Involvement of people with dementia in raising awareness and changing attitudes in a dementia friendly community pilot project', *Dementia*, 18: 2679–94.

Phillipson, L. and Hammond, A. (2018) 'More than talking: A scoping review of innovative approaches to qualitative research involving people with dementia', *International Journal of Qualitative Methods*, 17(1): 1609406918782784.

Phinney, A., Kelson, E., Baumbusch, J., O'Connor, D. and Purves, B. (2016) 'Walking in the neighbourhood: Performing social citizenship in dementia', *Dementia*, 15(3): 381–94.

Public Health Agency of Canada (2019) *A Dementia Strategy for Canada: Together We Aspire*, Government of Canada, Ottawa, available from: https://www.canada.ca/content/dam/phac-aspc/images/services/publications/diseases-conditions/dementia-strategy/National%20Dementia%20Strategy_ENG.pdf

Puurveen, G. and Phinney, A. (2019) 'Confronting the narrative of loss: Art and agency in dementia and dementia care', *BC Studies*, 202: 125–50.

Quinn, C., Toms, G., Anderson, D. and Clare, L. (2016) 'A review of self-management interventions for people with dementia and mild cognitive impairment', *Journal of Applied Gerontology*, 35(11): 1154–88.

Rahman, S. and Swaffer, K. (2018) 'Assets-based approaches and dementia-friendly communities', *Dementia*, 17: 131–7.

Reilly, S.T., Harding, A.J.E., Morbey, H., Ahmed, F. Williamson, P.R., Swarbrick, C., Leroi, I., Davies, L., Reeves, D., Holland, F., Hann, M. and Keady, J. (2020) 'What is important to people with dementia living at home? A set of core outcome items for use in the evaluation of non-pharmacological community-based health and social care interventions', *Age and Ageing*, 49(4): 664–71, available from: https://doi.org/10.1093/ageing/afaa015 [Accessed 15 April 2021].

Standing Senate Committee on Social Affairs, Science and Technology (2016) *Dementia in Canada: A national strategy for dementia-friendly communities: Ottawa*, available from: https://sencanada.ca/content/sen/committee/421/SOCI/Reports/SOCI_6thReport_DementiaInCanada-WEB_e.pdf

Statistics Canada (2016) *Census Profile 2016 Census*, Government of Canada, Ottawa, available from: https://www12.statcan.gc.ca/census-recensement/2016/dp-pd/prof/index.cfm?Lang=E

Ward, R., Clark, A., Campbell, S., Graham, B., Kullberg, A., Manji, K., Rummery, K. and Keady, J. (2018) 'The lived neighborhood: Understanding how people with dementia engage with their local environment', *International Psychogeriatrics*, 30(6): 867–80.

Weick, K. (1984) 'Small wins: Redefining the scale of social problems', *American Psychologist*, 39(1): 40–9.

Wiersma, E.C., McAiney, C., Loiselle, L., Hickman, K. and Harvey, D. (2016a) 'Shifting focus: Agency and resilience in a self-management programme for people living with dementia', in Clarke, C., Schwannauer, M., Taylor, J. and Rhynas, S. (eds) *Risk and Resilience: Global Learning Across the Age Span*, Edinburgh: Dunedin Academic Press.

Wiersma, E.C., O'Connor, D.L., Loiselle, L., Hickman, K., Heibein, B., Hounam, B., and Mann, J. (2016b) 'Creating space for citizenship: The impact of group structure on validating the voices of people with dementia', *Dementia*, 15(3): 414–33.

Wiersma, E.C. and Pedlar, A. (2008) 'The nature of relationships in alternative dementia care environments', *Canadian Journal on Aging*, 27: 101–8.

Windle, G., Joling, K.J., Howson-Griffiths, T., Woods, B., Jones, C.H., van de Ven, P.M., Newman, A. and Parkinson, C. (2018) 'The impact of a visual arts program on quality of life, communication, and well-being of people living with dementia: A mixed-methods longitudinal investigation', *International Psychogeriatrics*, 30(3): 409–23.

World Health Organization and Alzheimer Disease International (2012) *Dementia: A public health priority*, World Health Organization, available from: https://www.who.int/mental_health/publications/dementia_report_2012/en/

11

The good, the challenging and the supportive: mapping life with dementia in the community

Chris Brennan-Horley, Lyn Phillipson, Louisa Smith and Dennis Frost

Introduction

Developing bodies of work in interdisciplinary dementia research are engaging with concepts of place and spatiality as they relate to the everyday experience of living with dementia (Clarke and Bailey, 2016; Odzakovic et al, 2018). Rather than focus on the 'dis-abilities' of a person and their effect on navigation or wayfinding, these works have looked first to understand environmental barriers and to improve the enabling characteristics of environments – through features such as signage, pathways and distinctiveness (Mitchell and Burton, 2010). Building upon understanding the role of material geographies is work that engages with more progressive understandings of neighbourhoods as spaces of lived experience, belonging and relational ties (Ward et al, 2018; Clark et al, 2020). This evolving understanding of the vital importance of place and space for people with dementia is in contrast to a spatial literature where the relationship of people with dementia to space was pathologised – for example the reframing of the everyday practice of walking as a form of deviant wandering (Brittain et al, 2017). Rather than support mobility, a pathologising spatial lens problematises outdoor mobility for people with dementia as a health and safety risk and a social burden (MacAndrew et al, 2018). For those receiving a dementia diagnosis, notions like 'prescribed dis-engagement' (Swaffer, 2015) can foreclose possibilities for continuing involvement in the everyday spaces of community life. This prevalent narrative within the medicalised model sees dementia as a disease without a cure, with many medical practitioners accompanying diagnoses with instructions to abandon activities that are crucial to well-being and personhood and focus instead on end-of-life affairs and a potential trajectory of suffering.

People living with dementia have the right to freedom of movement and liberty and to be supported to maintain an 'activity space' (Hägerstrand, 1970) of regular social activities and movement within their neighbourhoods (Cahill 2018; Steele et al, 2019). These rights are being demanded through dementia activism and a closer alignment with the disability rights movement (Thomas and Milligan, 2018; Shakespeare et al, 2019). A new commitment to inclusion is also evident in some expressions of the international Dementia Friendly Communities (DFC) movement (Alzheimer's Disease International, 2017). In this context, there is a critical need for new ways to understand how a person with dementia engages with material activity space and neighbourhood; derives meaning from such places; and experiences agency and belonging through maintaining a physical presence in community spaces.

In this chapter we seek to contribute to this emerging and important topic by introducing qualitative mapping to dementia and neighbourhood research. We argue that involving people with dementia in mapping practices is not only productive for understanding their lived experience of traversing and being in community spaces, but also a constructive means to advocate for meaningful change.

Mapping: from the cartographic to the critical

Maps are deeply embedded and universal cultural practices that we engage with primarily to make spatial decisions (Stea et al, 1996). From viewing and engaging with map images perhaps as tactile objects (such as a tourist map or building office plan) or as digital media (such as Google maps routing a journey), maps and spatial technologies are an everyday part of our lives. Cartographic maps also have potent performative qualities, both recording and becoming political events that help to create the worlds they set out to document (Crampton, 2009; Rose-Redwood and Glass, 2014).

Mapping practices of spatial analysis and cartographic display have expanded in recent decades through Geographic Information Systems (GIS). GIS store, analyse and present geographic data and are particularly adept at visualising patterns within and between multiple digital inputs. In other words, GIS can create maps that overlay various layers of information, such as population health statistics, road networks and land use categories, permitting spatial analysis routines to run within and between layers.

As such, GIS support decisions around planning and governing space, producing tangible impacts across numerous social, economic and health spheres. Epidemiology and public health have used spatial analysis for hundreds of years to explain location-based relationships between population characteristics and health outcomes. Since GIS became widely available in the late 1990s, these fields have seen a rapid uptake of GIS capacity to understand and plan interventions for all manner of health issues, including infectious diseases, cancers and chronic conditions (Cromley and McLafferty, 2005). In the dementia context, Bagheri et al (2018) deployed GIS to understand the concentration and forecasting of dementia diagnoses to support health service planning, with an eye to placing key dementia services in those communities with the highest need. From an outdoor mobility standpoint, Wettstein et al (2015) used a combination of GPS tracking, GIS and multivariate statistics to create typologies of walking types among people with dementia.

The bulk of public health engagements with GIS fit within a spatial-analytic biomedical approach, that is, a reliance on spatial and statistical routines suitable for modelling, forecasting and visualising disease clustering; mapping population attributes that can indicate spatial patterns of health risks; and uncovering the geography of health disparities and access to services. However, interest is growing in deploying GIS as part of mixed methodological inquiries, where a plurality of methods can permit more nuanced understandings of a research problem over GIS data and methods alone (Kwan, 2002). This can be particularly helpful in research that seeks to illuminate the contextual role of place and neighbourhood in individual and small group health and well-being outcomes. Examples that have taken this approach include research on childhood obesity (Wridt, 2010); adolescent drug behaviour (Mennis et al, 2013); welfare-dependant families (Matthews et al, 2005); experiences of place for the over-70s (Milton et al, 2015); and social enterprise research (Farmer et al, 2020). These studies are beneficiaries of broader epistemic debates as to the nature of GIS that have successfully decoupled the technology from its supposed quantitative roots.

Following trenchant critique of GIS as quantitative and unsuitable for social and qualitative researchers (see Pickles, 1995), critical GIS scholars saw potential rather than foreclosure, forging ahead with alternate and productive engagements with GIS. These included Feminist GIS for visualising gendered axes of difference across time-space (Kwan, 2002) and a broad array of participatory GIS practices that sought to involve marginalised communities or groups in map making for their own ends and advocacy (Dunn, 2007; Elwood, 2008). Across the early 2000s, GIS began to be seen as a 'critical visual method' that can assist understanding of the spatiality of social processes (Kwan and Knigge, 2006, p 2001).

This potential is increasingly being realised by researchers and projects that adopt a Qualitative GIS stance. Qualitative GIS can be thought of as a mixed methods framework that bridges between analytical mappings and diverse qualitative ways of knowing. It recognises that all knowledge is partial, situated and complex (Elwood and Cope, 2009). Qualitative GIS can thus be integrated with a variety of data sources familiar to qualitative and ethnographic research (for example narrative text, audio, photo, video and sketches). These can be triangulated and combined with quantitative data for subsequent spatial visualisation. The analytical and visualisation capacities of GIS open spaces of possibility for project-specific mixes of data types and epistemologies to collide, often in productive and unforeseen ways (Brown and Knopp, 2008; Gibson et al, 2010).

Social health, dementia and space

The social health model of dementia (Huber et al, 2011; Vernooiji-Dassen and Jeon, 2016) recognises not only the contribution of individual capabilities, but also the importance of space and place as mediators of well-being within the everyday lives of people with dementia. A number of methods have been used to understand the role of place and its contribution to social health, including quantitative auditing for the presence of dementia design principles within community buildings (Fleming et al, 2017) and neighbourhood precincts (Su, 2013); and qualitative methods such as interviewing and walking interviews (Mitchell and Burton, 2010). Some of these have engaged with mapping in a limited way, for example in walk-around interviews as part of field notations (Ward et al, 2018); as an aide to communicating design principles which emerged as important to community mobility (Mitchell and Burton, 2010); or as a means for revealing important social networks across multiple scales (Clark et al, 2020). This work engages with and draws on spatial concepts and geographic language when analysing, synthesising and presenting findings. However, there is a reliance upon narrative approaches and textual representation, so while these modalities convey information about spatial relations, an opening remains to build upon textual accounts with rhetorically powerful cartographic images.

In the research we report upon, Qualitative GIS afforded new sense-making capacities about how people living with dementia use and move through urban space and where the barriers and possibilities lie to further social and spatial engagement. We now move to a detailed discussion of the mapping methods used to generate data with people with dementia before presenting results under three themes of *meaning*, *accessibility* and *change*. We then discuss the ways that mapping took on a performative role, productively intervening at specific junctures in the research process, gesturing toward the goal of a dementia-friendly community.

Generating spatial data with people with dementia and their carers in Kiama

Kiama is a local government municipality with a population of over 21,000 people (Australian Bureau of Statistics, 2014). The dispersed built form consists of a small downtown area surrounded by low-density suburbs of free-standing family homes. Kiama is an example of what is known in Australia as a 'sea-change' town. It is popular with retirees as a place to live out their senior years due to its attractive coastal location, village atmosphere and relative access to cities (Wollongong and Sydney are both accessible via a railway corridor). The larger Kiama State Electorate has a population of 69,000 people (Australian Bureau of Statistics, 2011). Due to the ageing demographic profile of the region, the number of people living with dementia in the State Electorate is projected to increase from the current 1,200 to almost 4,000 by 2050 (Australian Bureau of Statistics, 2012).

The Dementia Friendly Kiama project, which commenced as a partnership between the University of Wollongong, Dementia Australia and the local Kiama municipal council (Phillipson and Hall, 2020), was guided by its use of a Community Based Participatory Action Research framework (Israel et al, 1998). In the early stages of the project two governance groups were formed: a Dementia Advisory Group (consisting of people living with dementia and their carers); and a Dementia Alliance (including members of the Advisory Group, representatives from partner and other organisations, and interested individuals). Both of these groups have participated in the various cycles of formative and evaluative research and taken actions in response to create local change. These included increasing community awareness about dementia and local services, promoting understanding of the lived experience of dementia (in particular how they moved about and utilised community environments), reducing the stigma of dementia and improving the accessibility of the local environment (Phillipson et al, 2019).

As part of these cycles of research and action, we used two methods to generate qualitative spatial data: sketch mapping and crowdsourced maps.

Sketch mapping

Sketch maps are a paper map of a study area for participants to sketch and draw on while answering questions about that particular place (Boschmann and Cubbon, 2014). The sketching technique emerged from the mental map tradition that is carried out on a blank page, permitting an individual's cognitive map and sense of place to emerge through drawings of their favourite landmarks, ways and nodes (Lynch, 1960; Gieseking, 2013). Sketch maps extend upon mental mapping, as the base map, instead of a blank page, has features already drawn on it. This has a twofold impact on the resulting data. First, regarding elicitation, sketch maps encourage deep engagement with the base map, permitting participant and researcher to effectively place themselves in it, by orienting themselves against any map features (for example via the street network or by using the names or symbols representing physical or built landscape features). Second, the base map encourages relatively spatially accurate markings to be made in an additive fashion. Later georeferencing and conversion into GIS data 'lifts' and separates any markings made by participants from the underlying base map.

In 2014–15, local Kiama residents living with dementia and their carer partners were recruited to take part in dyadic sketch mapping interviews to explore their daily experiences of activities undertaken 'at home' and 'out and about' in the community. Participants were recruited through local council and community service groups. Prior to commencing interviews, all participants were provided with a written Participation Information Sheet. The details of the study were also verbally explained, with opportunities for people to ask direct questions to promote informed consent from the people with dementia. Written consent was obtained from both the person with dementia and their supporter/carer. Researchers also attended to verbal and behavioural indicators throughout to monitor the willingness and engagement of participants. Ethical approval for both was provided by the University Human Ethics Committee HE14/065.

Twelve interview dyads – each comprised of a participant with dementia and their care partner – were successfully recruited. Participants with dementia were aged between 60 and 84 years. Two had younger onset dementia. Seven of our participants living with dementia were female and five were male. All spoke English at home, and the majority lived in their own private homes or apartments with an informal care partner. Most (7 out of 12) of the care partners were in a married or de facto relationship with the person with dementia, one was a friend and two were adult children of the person with dementia. Ten out of 12 recalled they had been given a formal diagnosis of dementia and all of these had been diagnosed within the previous two years. Most could walk more than 500m without assistance and 8 out of 12 rated their overall quality of life as either good or very good.

All except one of the mapping interviews were conducted face to face in the participants' homes – the exception taking place in a local cafe. This approach promoted familiarity and comfort, avoided connotations of a clinical interview, and made use of environmental cues. The majority were conducted by two researchers. One acted as the primary interviewer of the person with dementia, with the second often interviewing the carer separately or taking notes or facilitating further discussion where appropriate. Interviews were audio recorded for later transcription. Sample questions from the interview guide included:

- What sort of things do you get up to during a typical week when you are 'out and about'?
- Where are the places you like to go? Are there any places you don't like to go?
- How does the environment support you to maintain the activities/ roles you are interested in? Where? What type of support do you require and from whom?
- Is there anything that could be done to support you in getting 'out and about' that would improve your quality of life?

Along with the traditional semi-structured interview technique, we produced two individual maps for each participant: one that represented their immediate local neighbourhood and another that represented the Kiama village centre (or high street). These were produced to reflect and provide a visual backdrop to the places and experiences that people were describing.

When used in interviews with people living with dementia, sketch mapping presented opportunities and pitfalls. Drawing and sketching during interviews can sometimes break down power relationships between researcher and participants, particularly for those less adept at expressing themselves verbally (Brennan-Horley et al, 2010). However, in our interviews, participants sometimes found it challenging to draw on sketch maps. Map reading and wayfinding can present particular challenges for some people with dementia (Mitchell and Burton, 2010). Researchers did provide some support around comprehending the maps when necessary, pointing to, questioning and drawing on participants' directions. Overall, the sketch maps grounded discussions about the everyday activity space of our participants – broadly, documenting and discussing places they travelled to and any underlying experiences of everyday mobilities.

As is regularly the case with sketch mapping research, the map became an active agent in the interview (Brennan-Horley and Gibson, 2009), drawing everyone into it as we crouched around to discuss living in Kiama. Figure 11.1 illustrates how we were collectively able to produce a map of where one interviewee went (green highlighter is shown in the digital version of this book), any places that were of particular importance (blue highlighter is shown in the digital version of this book) and places of avoidance or difficulty (pink highlighter is shown in the digital version of this book).

Crowdsourced mapping online

To scale the affordances of sketch mapping up to a wider cohort beyond our interviewees we also included a crowdsourced webmap into our data collection. This crowdsourced mapping phase occurred after preliminary analysis of the sketch mapping interviews. Indeed it was prompted by the Kiama Dementia Advisory Group, who, upon seeing the collective cartographic results of the sketch map interviews (refer to Figures 11.3 and 11.4), saw the potential in continuing to map their town and hopefully effecting change through sharing geospatial information among themselves and with government representatives.

In a crowdsourced model the power of the crowd is harnessed to provide geospatial information through a distributed webmap interface (Sui et al, 2013). Supported by funding from the Dementia Australia Research Foundation, a crowdsourced webmap was created on www. socialpinpoint.com and placed upon a project webpage we dubbed 'ourPlace'. Unlike the sketch map interviews, which targeted people living with dementia and their care partners or family, the ourPlace Kiama map invited contributions from anyone with internet access and an interest in the dementia-friendly issue. Users could access the crowdsourced map from a desktop computer or mobile device. Two different types of pins were available to the user to place upon the map. A blue pin for places they 'liked' or considered 'dementia friendly' and

Figure 11.1: A completed sketch map of Kiama Village

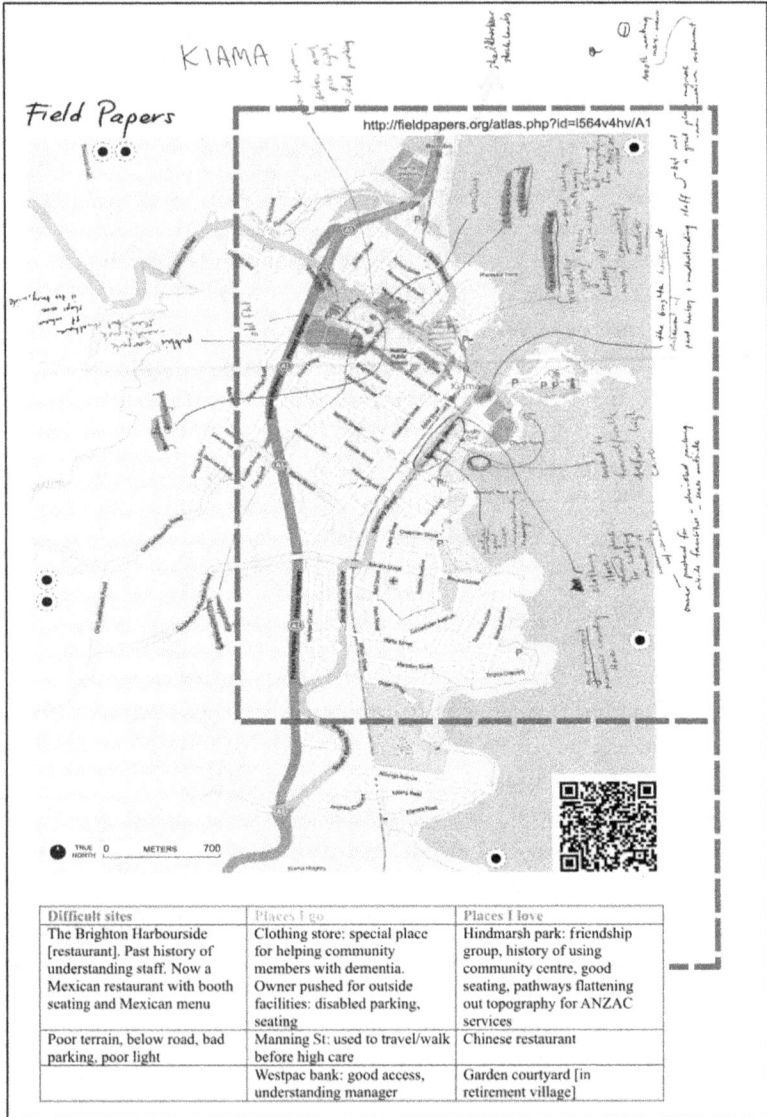

Difficult sites	Places I go	Places I love
The Brighton Harbourside [restaurant]. Past history of understanding staff. Now a Mexican restaurant with booth seating and Mexican menu	Clothing store: special place for helping community members with dementia. Owner pushed for outside facilities: disabled parking, seating	Hindmarsh park: friendship group, history of using community centre, good seating, pathways flattening out topography for ANZAC services
Poor terrain, below road, bad parking, poor light	Manning St: used to travel/walk before high care	Chinese restaurant
	Westpac bank: good access, understanding manager	Garden courtyard [in retirement village]

Note: Printed using www.fieldpapers.org. In addition to coloured highlights of places and paths, notes in black pen were made in real time by the interviewer to aid subsequent coding (Table 11.1 details comments from the boxed area). In line with a semi-structured interview, there were instances of data gathered about the past, of places participants went before their advancing condition affected involvement or access.

a yellow pin indicating 'ideas for action' or positive change. Once a pin was dropped a comment bubble permitted textual input, adding a photo, or responding or rating other submissions. Figure 11.2 shows a screen capture of the interface in action.

A total of 30 pins from 19 unique users were placed during the period of six months that the ourPlace map was promoted in Kiama; 19 of these represented places that people 'liked' or thought were 'dementia friendly' and there were 11 pins for 'ideas' for action. A subset of comments is provided in Table 11.1, alongside information on the type of user who provided the information.

Data analysis

Spatial data from the sketch map interviews were transferred into a GIS and interviews were transcribed. This data were analysed collectively and iteratively for triangulation and grounding purposes (Knigge and Cope, 2006). This supported rigour as we worked between the map sketches and transcription data, using each to inform the other, for example potentially moving incorrectly placed sketches based on written transcripts; providing more detail about key sites sketched on the map from the transcripts; or using spatial referents from sketches or the underlying base map to further understand the transcripts, especially in reference to particular sites. All paper sketch maps were scanned into digital .jpeg format and geo-referenced. This involves placing the digital image into the same coordinate space as the base map within the GIS, such that each sketch map sits exactly over the others. Responses to the three spatial interview questions were individually traced using a mouse and stored as three separate layers in a spatial database. This meant that all participant answers to the question 'where do you go in a typical week?' would now be stored together in a single composite layer, and so on. Corresponding attributes were populated for each response, such as location name, respondent and any contextual notes.

Processing data from the crowdsourced map was more straightforward. The socialpinpoint.com interface permitted all data (pin location, type, comments, responses, ratings and user type) to be extracted in a single spreadsheet. Incorporating this data into the spatial database was possible based upon the columns storing the latitude and longitude, with all attributes transferring directly over into the GIS.

A feature overlay was then used to visualise each of the sketch mapping questions. Overlays are perhaps the most popular GIS visualisation strategy as they draw upon our innate capabilities for pattern recognition and spatial reasoning (Pavlovskaya, 2006). This

Figure 11.2: The 'ourPlace' Kiama webmap interface

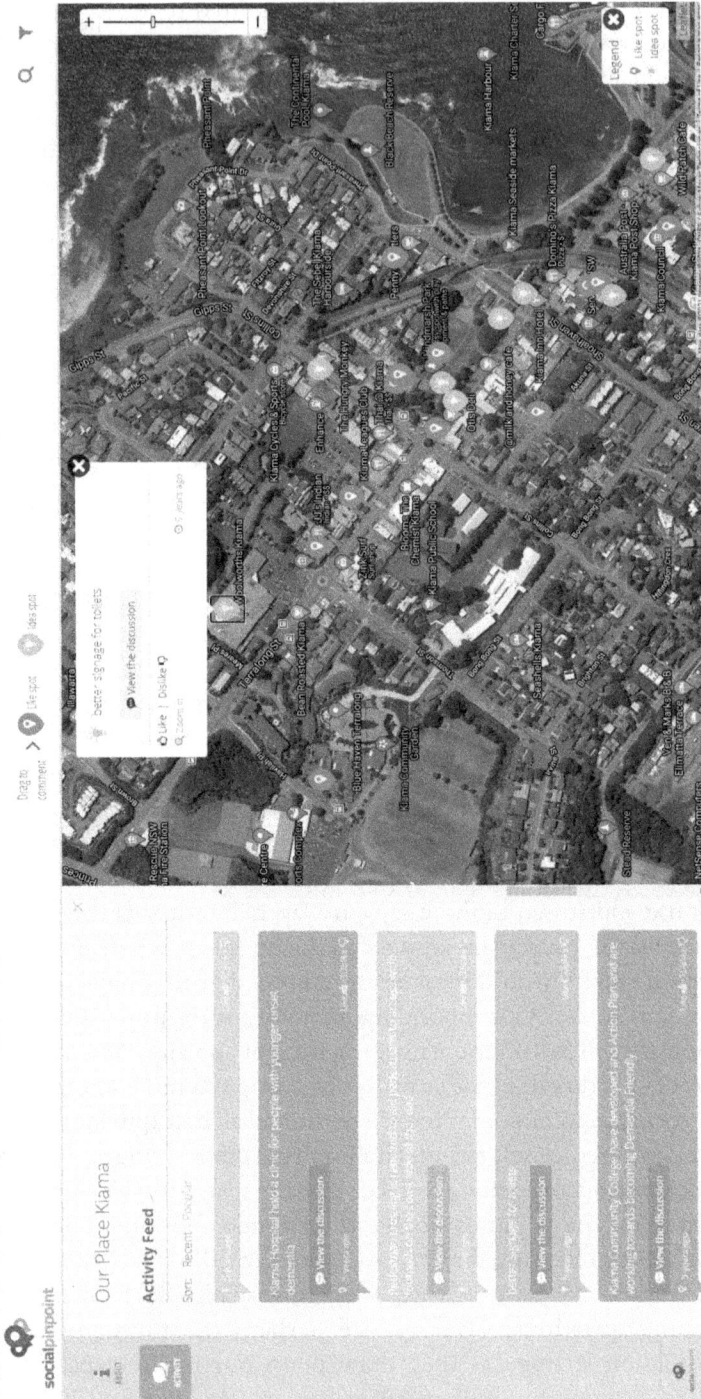

Note: As well as adding their own data, users could move around the map, inspect, rate and comment on other pins or look to the activity feed on the left.

Table 11.1: Sample of written responses from the Kiama 'ourPlace' crowdsourced webmap

Dementia friendly	User type
"The Sebel Hotel is a regular place I stay; and as a person living with dementia I find it reasonably dementia enabling. No garish carpets or loud music."	Community member living with dementia
"Friendly store."	Community member living with dementia
"Kiama Community Garden provides access to people of all ages and abilities to garden and socialise together. If you like gardening this is a great place for you."	Family carer or friend of someone living with dementia
"Good central all day parking, shaded on hot days. Walking access is smooth but steep."	Community member living with dementia
"Great to visit in summer time, has ramp and hand rail access. Ground is steady. Wheelchair access in pool area."	No information given
Ideas for action	**User type**
"Signage would be better at the end of the aisles not in each row so they can be viewed from either end of the store."	Family carer or friend of someone living with dementia
"Ambulance sign partially obscured by trees. Makes some navigation confusing as some of the toilet signs refer to 'next to the ambulance station' as part of the their direction."	Community member living with dementia
"Traffic-calming speed bump is confusing when trying to cross street. Should be marked out as a pedestrian crossing."	Support worker
"Street furniture for cafes partially block free footpath access."	Community member living with dementia
"My husband has dementia and limited mobility and enjoys a daily walk but needs to sit down several times. He has trouble with slopes and on the short slope next to boat ramp he has had several near-miss falls. The path along the harbour is flat and would be a better option to walk but there are no seats. I think several strategically placed seats would be beneficial."	Family carer or friend of someone living with dementia

process looks collectively at the spatial location of every participant response to a single question, essentially bringing all data for that single question together into one mapping frame. For example, across 12 interviews, the question 'where do you go?' resulted in 139 spatial features being separately traced from the paper maps and stored in the GIS. When brought together with a feature overlay, a sense of the spatial spread and any overlaps in participant responses quickly emerged (refer to Figure 11.3). To illustrate this concept numerically, ten markings were overlaid upon Kiama's 'Centro' shopping centre, meaning 80 per cent of our interviewees went there as part of their regular travels. Finally, interview transcriptions from the mapping interviews were uploaded into NVivo. This enabled thematic analysis and coding of textual data that enriched and provided additional context for interpretation alongside the maps.

Findings

We turn now to the results, looking at the data in terms of how the sketch maps and crowdsourced webmaps allowed us to think spatially about meaningful sites, the geography of accessibility and in supporting the Kiama Dementia Alliance to advocate for change.

Places of meaning

Participants in the sketch mapping interviews were asked some travel-related questions in the interview including: 'where do you go when you are out and about in a typical week in Kiama?' and 'which of these places are really enjoyable?' Broadly, a dichotomy emerged between travel to sites for leisure and enjoyment (cafes, restaurants, parks, community centres and places of worship) and visiting places to access essential services (grocery shops, banks and health services). In this data, places of leisure can be defined quite generally as places that supported participation in meaningful activities beyond what might nominally be called 'work'. These were sites where our participants undertook personal or community pursuits and provided purposeful opportunities for exercising agency through active engagement with self, others and the world (Iwasaki et al, 2018).

Figure 11.3 lets us see geospatial data from the dyadic interviews of people with dementia, illustrating their maintenance of a collective physical footprint in Kiama. In both frames, the feature overlay increases in darker shades where multiple spatial responses lined up. Our participants regularly visit sites across the entirety of the commercial zone. Concentrations emerged as they moved between key sites located predominantly within Kiama's town centre, adjacent public green space and dispersing out into coastal areas. Kiama's small, compact and walkable commercial zone maximised opportunities for social health, with meaningful sites either co-located or only a short distance apart. The overlay in Figure 11.3 illuminates the politics of social inclusion for people with dementia, pointing to a worldview where people with dementia are present in the material shared spaces (shops, parks, streets and so on) of community life. Figure 11.3 can thus be read as a performative act, documenting and presenting a collective spatial achievement that directly counters 'prescribed dis-engagement' narratives (Swaffer, 2015).

Additionally, Figure 11.3 highlights that instrumental and leisureful spaces are not necessarily spatially distinct. Indeed, these activities were often co-located. Both the mapping activity and the resulting collective visualisation allowed us to understand the multiple layers of meaning that mobility achieved. For example, Kiama's small Centro shopping centre, consisting of a grocery store and a small array of speciality shops, featured most prominently in the spatial data. But it was not solely an access point to essential services, as one participant living with dementia said:

'I love to go over the Centro here and, and it's ... everybody's very friendly and you can have a nice cup of coffee and that's what we did this afternoon. We met and we had a nice coffee there ... you go into Centro and they all say hello to you whether they know you or not. You know what I mean, and you can start up a few words like a beautiful day or something like that and you come home and think oh, I met so and so today.'

Figure 11.3: Places people with dementia go (left) vs places of special importance (right)

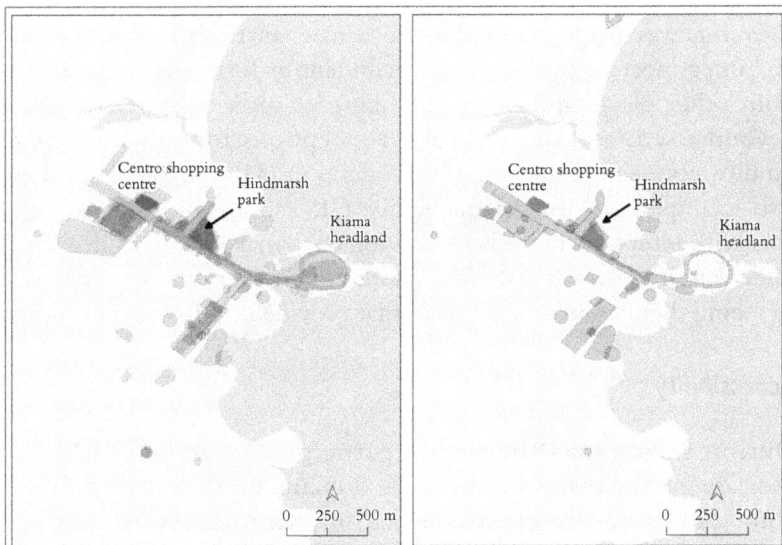

A visit to essential services became more meaningful because it provided opportunities to meet with relatives and also to 'bump into' other community members. Active engagement and exercising of personal agency through interactions with shopkeepers, health professionals and the broader community meant our participants contributed to their social health, simply by participating in the everyday social life of Kiama.

Our data also pointed to the important role of memory of past experiences from other places played in the simple joyful act of sitting down and watching community activity unfold. To illustrate, the aquatic centre, located across the road from the Blue Haven retirement village, also features a small cafe. One carer spoke about her recently deceased father who lived with dementia and was a regular visitor to the centre before his passing:

> 'He'd often go over to the Leisure Centre, like, I think independence, that's where he'd buy like a little coffee and he'd often sit and have a coffee and think that he'd had a bit of an outing. I think he liked ... again there's a lot of activity there, you know, children jumping into pools, people swimming. He'd spend a lot of time, he was into ... he was a Bondi, you know the Bondi Icebergs [Sydney's world-famous winter swimming club] in his younger days, and a lot of time at Bondi Beach at the gym and things like that.'

Meaning was made at the aquatic centre relationally (Clark et al, 2020), connecting that site to pivotal identity-formation experiences from other places and times. Thinking of space relationally moves beyond fixed, asocial and scalar conceptions towards notions of fluidity, connection and social reproduction (Massey, 2005). In these two examples we see the qualitative GIS combination of mapping data with interview narratives allowing us to make the transition from understanding sites as individual nodes in an everyday activity space to seeing them as relational places that provide multilayered meaning.

Accessibility

During sketch map interviews participants were also asked to indicate places that were perhaps difficult or that they avoided. Difficult places were often couched in terms relating to problems with physical accessibility when attempting to move through Kiama's built environment. Kiama has numerous characteristics that promote walkability. Most of the meaningful sites were within walking distance of each other, even for those requiring mobility aids. Footpaths are provided on both sides of the main street and the presence of a rail station close to the centre of town helped make Kiama accessible to nearby urban centres. Yet the topographic story was mixed. The main street was deemed generally manageable as it is on a reasonably gentle slope. This permitted residents from the nearby Blue Haven retirement village, some of whom live with dementia, to easily move down into the main commercial zone with its multiple options for social connection. However, the residential parts of Kiama range from undulating to quite steep only a couple of streets back from the main road. These were understandably difficult to access for those with mobility issues, who would avoid using these streets, and were indicated by multiple respondents in Figure 11.4, in response to the question of difficult places or sites of avoidance.

While a simple topographic map can provide information about physical accessibility, the sketch and crowdsourced maps allowed users to indicate physical locations at the same time as providing a contextual narrative. This allowed for the overlay of information about social and cognitive accessibility. For example, shops where staff were more helpful and understanding were deemed more accessible for people with dementia and they would continue to frequent those over others. One particular Chinese restaurant was mentioned and mapped by multiple interviewees. Situated only a stone's throw from Kiama's Blue Haven retirement village and accessible via a clearly marked, raised pedestrian crossing at its front door, it was regularly visited and perceived as very welcoming to older Kiama residents and those living with dementia. One carer noted:

> 'I think it's a lot to do with the owner of the Chinese restaurant and how welcoming he is. It's not flash inside, in the interior, there's no view, but he makes them welcome and makes [people] feel valued. There's tablecloths on the tables which I think older people still like those things so it's homely. It's a homely atmosphere. He also does a lot of deliveries to Blue Haven [retirement village].'

A caring attitude and familiar decor were prioritised over aesthetics. This speaks to the important role that customer service attitudes and training initiatives that focus on increasing dementia awareness could have upon perceptions of social inclusiveness. When considering accessibility and how well community members living with dementia can manage when out and about, interpersonal encounters can be as important for the experience of place as qualities relating to the accessibility, proximity or comfort afforded or constrained by the physical environment. Qualitative mapping that blends material location with narrative permitted this understanding to emerge.

The usefulness of qualitative GIS visualisation to this research was how it enabled us to see, in one frame, different kinds of information about places that might at first seem contradictory. This was particularly stark, for example, when we juxtaposed meaningful places with difficult ones. As shown in Figure 11.4, many of the places where our participants experienced access difficulties were also the most meaningful and enjoyable. Comparing the results to the different questions with a spatial overlay allowed this story to emerge. The good, the challenging and the supportive were intermingled.

People living with dementia are challenged daily to contend with the material environment, the presence or absence of social and physical supports and their ability to adapt. These factors intermingle in very personal ways to shape their experience of place. Our interviewees used a spectrum of coping strategies: they avoided difficult places at particular times like busy weekends or public holidays, received help

Figure 11.4: Places of difficulty/avoidance (left) and overlaid with meaningful places (right)

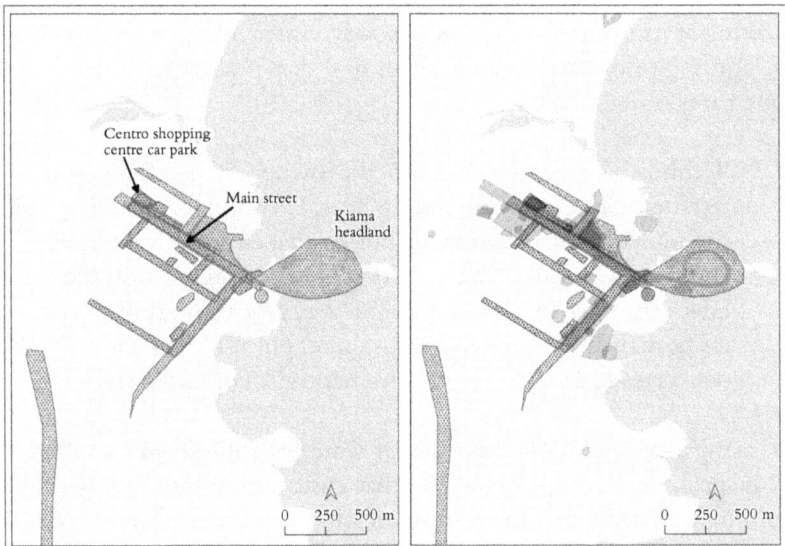

from others where possible, avoided the place altogether or continued to traverse the downtown area to get to meaningful places even though the journey presented risk.

ourPlace: mapping for change

Across the research process, the crowdsourced map offered the greatest possibility to open a dialogue between our research participants and decision makers/managers of the urban environment. Given that maintaining the ability to move beyond home and interact socially with others in community settings is central to social health (Dröes et al, 2016), the crowdsourced map identified 'Ideas for action' that, if acted upon, could make problematic features within specific places more manageable and accessible.

Of all the pins placed on the Kiama map during its six months of active promotion, just over one third of these contained 'Ideas for action' pins. The majority promoted ideas for improvements to particular footpaths, kerbsides, pedestrian crossings, places for signage, car parking and public toilets (refer to Table 11.1 for emblematic examples). While the general focus of these issues may have been expected, what was not anticipated was that being able to identify specific places for action empowered the members of the Kiama Dementia Alliance. As part of the Alliance regular monthly meetings, postings from the ourPlace Kiama webmap were reviewed (refer to Figure 11.5). This map aided the transformation from a general discussion about 'how to make Kiama more dementia friendly' to discussions that were grounded in accountabilities and support for making the places that had been pinned better. Rather than face the impossible task of 'improving all environments', council officials were instead enabled to raise specific and manageable work orders with the relevant departments to fix specific instances of, for example, signage for public toilets, kerb repairs and extra seating along certain footpaths.

The specific dialogue enabled by the pins on the map also uncovered areas that were beyond the remit for local action – and required advocacy with other agencies – for example with the state government, which had responsibility for crosswalks on the main road. In all of this, the webmap grounded participants' pins and comments in tangible elements of the built environment that caused issues, while simultaneously acting as a conduit, communicating the lived experience of people with dementia to decision makers.

Figure 11.5: 'Ideas for action' pins from the 'ourPlace' crowdsourced webmap, labelled by type of issue raised

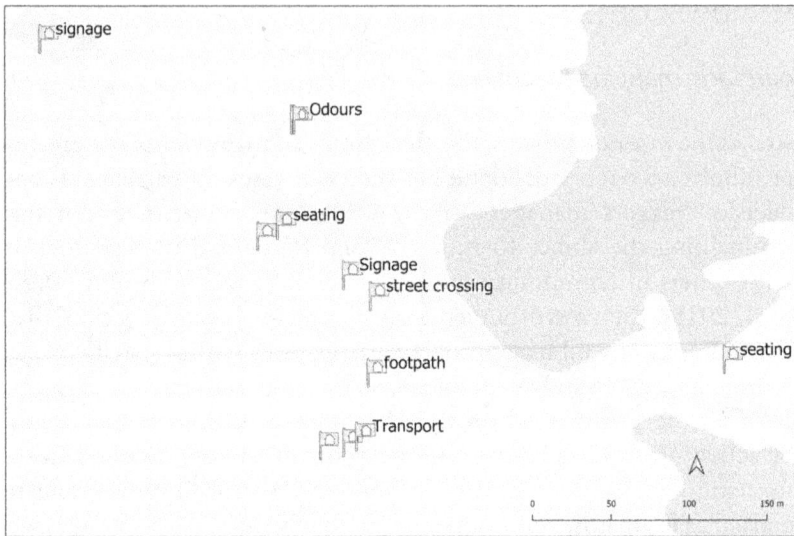

Conclusion

To our knowledge, this is the first study that has deployed qualitative GIS with people with dementia to understand their experience in a community setting. In this chapter we proposed the potential value of qualitative GIS to extend upon place-based and geographic/spatial concepts that inflect the more text-based qualitative social health research on dementia and neighbourhood environments. Our experience of mapping in the town centre of Kiama, was that qualitative GIS, with its blend of cartographic and textual narratives, brought fresh perspectives on how people living with dementia use and move through urban space and where the barriers and possibilities lie to further social and spatial engagement.

Qualitative mapping provided us with an additional means to understand both the complexity and dynamism of our participants' spatial experiences. Specifically, it captured complex and contradictory experiences of multiple individuals in one two-dimensional field, in a way that written forms of qualitative research are less adept at doing. Comprehending spoken or written words is a more cognitively demanding task than consuming images, as our pre-attentive visuospatial cortex processes images before cognition occurs (Ware, 2010). While qualitative interviews, walk-arounds and ethnographies can and do capture spatial complexities and contradictions, the maps – as visual images – rapidly revealed Euclidean (distance-based) spatial relationships, especially across our research cohort via the overlay method, making known, for instance, that meaningful sites and inaccessible sites were interwoven and overlapping. Place-based literature, which relies solely on written accounts of walk-arounds or interviews, while rich, potentially misses an opportunity to convey insightful geospatial relationships. Qualitative GIS can thus potentially generate new knowledge and rapid understanding about the experience of living with dementia in the community.

Across the research process we noticed the performative capacities of mapping effectively stepping in at four key junctures. First, during interviews with people with dementia and their care partners, the map had guiding qualities: grounding discussions upon material sites, generating qualitative contextual information about what took place there and functioning as an aide memoire for other sites that may otherwise have been missed. Second, without the map data, we as researchers would have found it difficult to 'see' the ways in which meaningful and unmanageable spaces overlapped across our participants. The output maps in Figures 11.3 and 11.4 thus have transformative potential for interdisciplinary dementia research and activism to counter pathologising narratives of disengagement. These particular maps perform by visually carving out space for people with dementia as part of the community, generating meaning in the everyday tasks that stigmatising perspectives consider overly challenging or unachievable (Phillipson et al, 2012). Third, the maps fired the imagination of the Dementia Advisory Group, who clearly saw the advocacy potential that mapping could have, pushing us to launch the ourPlace webmap so they could continue mapping. This is in line with counter-mapping and participatory GIS, where the spatial knowledge and expertise of marginalised communities can be harnessed to create their own cartographies, with the outputs being brought to bear upon governance and planning to create more inclusive communities. Finally, and following on from the previous point, this performative power was realised through the crowdsourced map as a catalysing agent for change. Revealing actionable anchor points in the landscape with a map prompted decision makers to act. Across these four moments we follow Corner's (1999) conceptualisation of maps as having rhizomatic qualities – that is, mapping practices have diverse entry points and exits that create new and multiple possibilities for unfolding action. In Kiama, our maps displayed agency numerous times, assisting in bringing a more dementia-friendly Kiama into being.

Our final point is that qualitative GIS exposed Kiama as neither 'dementia friendly' nor 'unfriendly'. Rather, meaningful sites and gradations of accessibility intersected irregularly across the town. This reflects the mix of capabilities and desires of our small cohort only and as such, the geographies revealed in our qualitative mappings are only ever partial and subjective. However, they do hint at the uncomfortable possibility that even if material or social aspects are altered for the better for one person, they may remain challenging, meaningless or exclusionary for another. Dementia-friendly communities need to remain alive to the diversity of spatial experiences and meanings that collectively make up the rhythms of everyday life. Our qualitative mapping methods show there may well be areas where certain elements line up, cluster or clash. Mapping this diversity of everyday encounters and experiences can hopefully set the stage for productive discussions around how best to work through those issues in ways that are as inclusive as possible for people living with dementia to remain active community members.

References

Alzheimer's Disease International (2017) 'Dementia friendly communities. Global developments 2nd edition', available from: https://www.alzint.org/u/dfc-developments.pdf [Accessed 9 January 2020].

Australian Bureau of Statistics (2011) 'Census QuickStats: Kiama State Electoral Divisions', available from: http://www.censusdata.abs.gov.au/census_services/getproduct/census/2011/quickstat/SED10038?opendocument&navpos=220 [Accessed 16 September 2020].

Australian Bureau of Statistics (2012) 'Australian social trends: People identified as having dementia or Alzheimer's disease', available from: https://www.abs.gov.au/AUSSTATS/abs@.nsf/Lookup/4102.0Main+Features50Dec+2012 [Accessed 20 January 2021].

Australian Bureau of Statistics (2014) 'Kiama Region data summary', available from: http://stat.abs.gov.au/itt/r.jsp?RegionSummary&region=14400&dataset=ABS_REGIONAL_LGA&geoconcept=REGION&datasetASGS=ABS_REGIONAL_ASGS&datasetLGA=ABS_REGIONAL_LGA&regionLGA=REGION&regionASGS=REGION [Accessed 20 January 2021].

Bagheri, N., Wangdi, K., Cherbuin, N. and Anstey, K.J. (2018) 'General practice clinical data help identify dementia hotspots: A novel geospatial analysis approach', *Journal of Alzheimer's Disease*, 61(1): 125–34.

Boschmann, E.E. and Cubbon, E. (2014) 'Sketch maps and qualitative GIS: Using cartographies of individual spatial narratives in geographic research', *The Professional Geographer*, 66(2): 236–48.

Brennan-Horley, C. and Gibson, C. (2009) 'Where is creativity in the city? Integrating qualitative and GIS methods', *Environment and Planning A: Economy and Space*, 41(11): 2595–614.

Brennan-Horley, C., Luckman, S., Gibson, C. and Willoughby-Smith, J. (2010) 'GIS, ethnography, and cultural research: Putting maps back into ethnographic mapping', *The Information Society*, 26(2): 92–103.

Brittain, K., Degnen, C., Gibson, G., Dickinson, C. and Robinson, L. (2017) 'When walking becomes wandering: Representing the fear of the fourth age', *Sociology of Health and Illness*, 39(2): 270–84.

Brown, M. and Knopp, L. (2008) 'Queering the map: The productive tensions of colliding epistemologies', *Annals of the Association of American Geographers*, 98(1): 40–58.

Cahill, S. (2018) *Dementia and Human Rights*, Bristol: Policy Press.

Clark, A., Campbell, S., Keady, J., Kullberg, A., Manji, K., Rummery, K. and Ward, R. (2020) 'Neighbourhoods as relational places for people living with dementia', *Social Science and Medicine*, 252: 112927.

Clarke, C.L. and Bailey, C. (2016) 'Narrative citizenship, resilience and inclusion with dementia: On the inside or on the outside of physical and social places', *Dementia*, 15(3): 434–52.

Corner, J. (1999) 'The agency of mapping: Speculation, critique and invention', in Cosgrove, D. (ed) *Mappings*, London: Reaktion Books, pp 213–52.

Crampton, J.W. (2009) 'Cartography: Performative, participatory, political', *Progress in Human Geography*, 33(6): 840–48.

Cromley, E.K. and McLafferty, S. (2005) *GIS and Public Health*, New York: Guilford Press.

Dröes, R.M., Chattat, R., Diaz, A., Gove, D., Graff, M., Murphy, K., Verbeek, H., Vernooij-Dassen, M., Clare, L., Johannessen, A., Roes, M., Verhey, F. and Charras, K. (2016) 'Social health and dementia: A European consensus on the operationalization of the concept and directions for research and practice', *Aging and Mental Health*, 21(1): 4–17.

Dunn, C.E. (2007) 'Participatory GIS – a people's GIS?', *Progress in Human Geography*, 31(5): 616–37.

Elwood, S. (2008) 'Grassroots groups as stakeholders in spatial data infrastructures: Challenges and opportunities for local data development and sharing', *International Journal of Geographical Information Science*, 22(1): 71–90.

Elwood, S. and Cope, M. (2009) 'Introduction: Qualitative GIS: Forging mixed methods through representations, analytical innovations, and conceptual engagements', in Cope, M. and Elwood, S. (eds) *Qualitative GIS*, London: Sage Publications, pp 1–12.

Farmer, J., Kamstra, P., Brennan-Horley, C., De Cotta, T., Roy, M., Barraket, J., Munoz, S.A. and Kilpatrick, S. (2020) 'Using micro-geography to understand the realisation of wellbeing: A qualitative GIS study of three social enterprises', *Health and Place*, 62: 1–11.

Fleming, R., Bennett, K., Preece, T. and Phillipson, L. (2017) 'The development and testing of the dementia friendly communities environment assessment tool (DFC EAT)', *International Psychogeriatrics*, 29(2): 303–11.

Gibson, C., Brennan-Horley, C. and Warren, A. (2010) 'Geographic information technologies for cultural research: Cultural mapping and the prospects of colliding epistemologies', *Cultural Trends*, 19(4): 325–48.

Gieseking, J.J. (2013) 'Where we go from here: The mental sketch mapping method and its analytic components', *Qualitative Inquiry*, 19(9): 712–24.

Hägerstrand, T. (1970) 'What about people in regional science?', *Papers of the Regional Science Association*, 24(1): 6–21.

Huber, M., Knottnerus, J.A., Green, L., Horst, H.V.D., Jadad, A.R., Kromhout, D., Leonard, B., Lorig, K., Loureiro, M.I., Meer, J.W.M.V.D., Schnabel, P., Smith, R., Weel, C.V. and Smid, H. (2011) 'How should we define health?', *British Medical Journal*, 343: d4163.

Israel, B.A., Schulz, A.J., Parker, E.A. and Becker, A.B. (1998) 'Review of community-based research: Assessing partnership approaches to improve public health', *Annual Review of Public Health*, 19(1): 173–202.

Iwasaki, Y., Messina, E.S. and Hopper, T. (2018) 'The role of leisure in meaning-making and engagement with life', *The Journal of Positive Psychology*, 13(1): 29–35.

Knigge, L. and Cope, M. (2006) 'Grounded visualization: Integrating the analysis of qualitative and quantitative data through grounded theory and visualization', *Environment and Planning A: Economy and Space*, 38(11): 2021–37.

Kwan, M.P. (2002) 'Feminist visualization: Re-envisioning GIS as a method in feminist geographic research', *Annals of the Association of American Geographers*, 92(4): 645–61.

Kwan, M.P. and Knigge, L. (2006) 'Doing qualitative research using GIS: An oxymoronic endeavour?', *Environment and Planning A: Economy and Space*, 38: 1999–2002.

Lynch, K. (1960) *The Image of the City*, Cambridge: MIT Press.

MacAndrew, M., Schnitker, L., Shepherd, N. and Beattie, E. (2018) 'People with dementia getting lost in Australia: Dementia related missing person reports in the media', *Australasian Journal on Ageing*, 37(3): E97–E103.

Massey, D. (2005) *For Space*, London: Sage Publications.

Matthews, S.A., Detwiler, J.E. and Burton, L.M. (2005) 'Geo-ethnography: Coupling geographic information analysis techniques with ethnographic methods in urban research', *Cartographica: The International Journal for Geographic Information and Geovisualization*, 40(4): 75–90.

Mennis, J., Mason, M.J. and Cao, Y. (2013) 'Qualitative GIS and the visualization of narrative activity space data', *International Journal of Geographical Information Science*, 27(2): 267–91.

Milton, S., Pliakas, T., Hawkesworth, S., Nanchahal, K., Grundy, C., Amuzu, A., Casas, J.P. and Lock, K. (2015) 'A qualitative geographical information systems approach to explore how older people over 70 years interact with and define their neighbourhood environment', *Health and Place*, 36: 127–33.

Mitchell, L. and Burton, E. (2010) 'Designing dementia-friendly neighbourhoods: Helping people with dementia to get out and about', *Journal of Integrated Care*, 18(6): 11–18.

Odzakovic, E., Hellström, I., Ward, R. and Kullberg, A. (2018) '"Overjoyed that I can go outside": Using walking interviews to learn about the lived experience and meaning of neighbourhood for people living with dementia', *Dementia*, available from: https://doi.org/10.1177/1471301218817453 [Accessed 15 April 2021].

Pavlovskaya, M. (2006) 'Theorizing with GIS: A tool for critical geographies?' *Environment and Planning A: Economy and Space*, 38(11): 2003–20.

Phillipson, L. and Hall, D (2020) 'Dementia Illawarra Website', *Dementia Friendly Kiama*, available from: http://dementiaillawarra.com/dementia-friendly-kiama/ [Accessed 20 January 2021].

Phillipson, L., Hall, D., Cridland, E., Fleming, R., Brennan-Horley, C., Guggisberg, N., Frost, D. and Hasan, H. (2019) 'Involvement of people with dementia in raising awareness and changing attitudes in a dementia friendly community pilot project', *Dementia*, 18(7–8): 2679–94.

Phillipson, L., Magee, C., Jones, S., Skladzien, E. and Cridland, E. (2012) 'Exploring dementia and stigma beliefs: A pilot study of Australian adults aged, 40–65', *Alzheimer's Australia*, available from: https://www.dementia.org.au/sites/default/files/Stigma_Report.pdf [Accessed 20 January 2021].

Pickles, J. (1995) *Ground Truth: The Social Implications of Geographic Information Systems*, New York: Guilford Press.

Rose-Redwood, R. and Glass, M.R. (2014) 'Introduction: Geographies of performativity', in Glass, M. and Rose-Redwood, R. (eds) *Performativity, Politics, and the Production of Social Space*, London: Routledge, pp 1–34.

Shakespeare, T., Zeilig, H. and Mittler, P. (2019) 'Rights in mind: Thinking differently about dementia and disability', *Dementia*, 18(3): 1075–88.

Stea, D., Blaut J.M. and Stephens J. (1996) 'Mapping as a cultural universal', in Portugali, J. (ed) *The Construction of Cognitive Maps. GeoJournal Library, vol 32*, Dordrecht: Springer, pp 345–60.

Steele, L., Swaffer, K., Phillipson, L. and Fleming, R. (2019) 'Questioning segregation of people living with dementia in Australia: An international human rights approach to care homes', *Laws*, 8(3): 1–26.

Su, J. (2013) 'Built for Dementia: Urban Design Analysis for Dementia-Friendly Communities' [unpublished thesis], San Jose State University, available from: https://scholarworks.sjsu.edu/cgi/viewcontent.cgi?article=1317&context=etd_projects [Accessed 9 January 2020].

Sui, D., Goodchild, M. and Elwood, S. (2013) 'Volunteered geographic information, the exaflood, and the growing digital divide', in Sui, D., Elwood, S. and Goodchild, M. (eds) *Crowdsourcing Geographic Knowledge*, Dordrecht: Springer, pp 1–12.

Swaffer, K. (2015) 'Dementia and prescribed disengagement', *Dementia*, 14(1): 3–6.

Thomas, C. and Milligan, C. (2018) 'Dementia, disability rights and disablism: Understanding the social position of people living with dementia', *Disability and Society*, 33(1): 115–31.

Vernooij-Dassen, M. and Jeon, Y.H. (2016) 'Social health and dementia: The power of human capabilities', *International Psychogeriatrics*, 28(5): 701–3.

Ward, R., Clark, A., Campbell, S., Graham, B., Kullberg, A., Manji, K., Rummery, K. and Keady, J. (2018) 'The lived neighborhood: Understanding how people with dementia engage with their local environment', *International Psychogeriatrics*, 30(6): 867–80.

Ware, C. (2010) *Visual Thinking for Design*, Burlington: Morgan Kaufman.

Wettstein, M., Wahl H.-W., Shoval N., Auslander G., Oswald F. and Heinik J. (2015) 'Identifying mobility types in cognitively heterogeneous older adults based on GPS-tracking: What discriminates best?', *Journal of Applied Gerontology*, 34(8): 1001–27.

Wridt, P. (2010) 'A qualitative GIS approach to mapping urban neighborhoods with children to promote physical activity and child-friendly community planning', *Environment and Planning B: Planning and Design*, 37(1): 129–47.

12

Growing back into community: changes through life with dementia

Dennis Frost

Prior to my diagnosis my involvement in community was centred around my extended family and work and work colleagues. Like many people, my family is spread over a large geographic area and meaningful interaction involves physical and social contact. This has necessitated regular travel by private car. Private transport provides a needed degree of flexibility and control that is lacking from public transport. Social interaction within my local community was limited to a small circle of friends who were predominately work colleagues.

Then came my diagnosis. In mid-2013 at the age of 59 I was diagnosed with younger onset dementia. As part of my diagnosis I was given three to six years to live and told that I should retire as soon as possible. I soon began to experience the stigmas associated with dementia that are often the result of people's misconceived stereotypes around dementia. My GP also advised me not to tell anyone I has frontotemporal dementia, but to say that I had frontotemporal degeneration. I didn't understand why she would advise this, but later realised it was a strategy to avoid the stigmas associated with dementia. I was also advised I either had to stop driving or have a driving test. However, it was both expensive and stressful to undergo a 'fitness to drive' assessment, just to prove I could still drive. So it felt like there were obstacles being put in the way of me continuing to do the things that were important to me. As I finished work my world of social interactions diminished and my interactions with the broader community contracted. What I experienced I later realised was best described as 'prescribed disengagement' (Swaffer, 2015), being advised to withdraw from 'normal' life, get my affairs in order and prepare to die. My broad group of social contacts contracted to a few friends and family. My interactions within my local neighbourhood became those oriented around doing 'essential tasks' such as grocery shopping and medical appointments – a model that could have been the prototype of 'social isolation' in today's world of COVID-19.

After about 18 months of this contracting social world, I was invited to attend an early public meeting of what was to become the 'Dementia Friendly Kiama Project'. This meeting was aimed at informing and inviting people living with dementia and their care partners to become involved in the project, forming a Dementia Advisory Group. The key speaker at this meeting was Kate Swaffer, a person who herself was living with younger onset dementia. I still remember a key message in her presentation – that having dementia does not mean that you are incapable of taking an active and leading role in the community. This point marked a change and the slow re-expansion of my social world. First, just travelling to the Dementia Friendly Kiama Advisory Group and Dementia Alliance meetings meant a reopening of the physical world to me and supported my venturing into an expanded local community. My world expanded because, like many of the people involved in the project, I lived outside the Kiama township – so my sense of neighbourhood got a whole lot bigger. As a group of individuals with diverse backgrounds and differing needs with our different forms of dementia, we soon began to meet informally and started not only to influence positive change, but also to experience the benefits of it. We later learned that our Kiama Dementia Advisory Group was one of the first such groups formed in the world to work with a local community rather than at a national level (Dementia Alliance International, 2016). At this time, and through this expanding larger social circle, I was introduced to the Dementia Alliance International (DAI). This newly formed group was an international alliance of people living with dementia and aimed to be a global voice for all with dementia. The DAI began a series of regular online social groups, and involvement in these meetings soon introduced me to an international group of peers, some of whom have had 20 years' personal experience living with dementia. These regular social meetings expanded my sense of community from local to global. Indeed, it has often been expressed by members of this group that they feel more connected to this virtual community than they do to their own local community.

As the Dementia Friendly Kiama project gained exposure there were many invitations for the project to be presented at conferences. These offers were accepted on the condition that two people would present, a representative of the Alliance and a member of the Dementia Advisory Group. I was fortunate to often be a co-presenter at these conferences. As such it was the first time that I had attended a conference in this role and it presented a stimulating challenge. Over a period of 18 months I co-presented the project at several state-based

Aged Care conferences and to several communities planning their own dementia-friendly initiatives.

I was then invited to be plenary speaker at the 2016 Alzheimer's Disease International annual conference in Budapest. Here I met many people who were part of an international community of dementia advocates. Most of these people were members of the DAI and living with dementia. These individuals exposed me more to the diverse abilities of people living with Dementia and grew my community involvement to a global scale.

This opportunity for overseas travel was a surprise. In the early 1980s I had travelled several times to the US as part of my career as a petroleum geophysicist and then again a few years later to Europe for a holiday that marked a major change in my career path. After my diagnosis I did not think I would ever be likely to travel by air again, let alone internationally. It also proved a point of interest to my former colleagues, who were now envious of my international travel and active participation at international conferences. Planning for this travel also led me to ask questions about end-of-life planning and therefore we as a family organised wills and power of attorney documents. I even planned the location where I wish my ashes to be spread.

About this time Alzheimer's Australia began to redesign its Dementia Friendly Community and Dementia Friends programme. I became a member of its National Advisory Group to contribute insights learned from the Kiama Project. This also introduced me to a national network of like-minded individuals. I got to share with them what was important in my neighbourhood and community. And they shared with me about theirs.

I was then invited to the 2017 Alzheimer's Disease International conference held in Kyoto, Japan to present the Kiama Dementia Friendly project to a Dementia Friendly Communities Workshop. I was the only person living with dementia presenting at this important workshop. This surprised me and I told the audience that any dementia-friendly initiatives that didn't involve and respect the input from community members living with dementia was tokenistic and doomed to ultimate failure. These comments I believe were well received by most of the audience.

In 2018 the Dementia Friendly Kiama project decided that we would develop and deliver our own dementia awareness presentations to the community. We have now delivered over ten of these presentations to the public and community groups. Recently I was asked to present similar material to The Engineeering Design Institute – London

(TEDI) summer school. It is empowering to know that work I do for our local community is also of benefit to people to use worldwide and is hopefully helping individuals shape their local neighbourhoods to be more dementia friendly.

I was also becoming more involved in participating in research projects. The more connections I made, the bigger my social network, the more research projects I became aware of. As my involvement increased so did my understanding of some of the hurdles the research community had to overcome. The first I became aware of was the difficulty of locating people willing to participate. This seemed strange as currently there are almost half a million people living with dementia in Australia and over 28,000 of us have been diagnosed with younger onset dementia. In 2018 I was again invited to be involved in a national conference. This time I was invited by the Alzheimer's Disease Association of Singapore to both present at their national conference and to view and discuss their developing Dementia Friendly Communities programme.

While participating in the Kyoto conference I witnessed a presentation of the 'Join Dementia Research' project in the UK and so it came as no surprise a few months later when I was invited to become involved as an advisor on a panel for what has now become 'Step Up For Dementia', a programme modelled on the UK project, but heavily modified for Australia, that aims to connect willing participants with worthy research projects.

More recently, my involvement has grown from being a participant in research projects to being involved in contributing to the defining of the scope and objectives of projects, designing and evaluating methodologies and even helping to inform human ethics committees about the experience of living with dementia (Phillipson and Frost, 2020).

This level of involvement has now meant that I have a sense of achievement. In 1973 I began my studies at the University of Wollongong, graduating five years later with a BSc (Hons) and Dip Ed Forty years later I have returned to share my experiences with life and to give back to that community.

Through the connections made with these projects my social and physical world has expanded and my sense of community has grown to well beyond what it was after my initial diagnosis in 2013. I have learned a lot along this path and can attest that while dementia is a debilitating condition it does offer insights that would otherwise be missed and is not all bad.

References

Dementia Alliance International (2016) *The Human Rights of People Living with Dementia: From Rhetoric to Reality*, p 9, available from: https://www.dementiaallianceinternational.org/wp-content/uploads/2016/05/Human-Rights-for-People-Living-with-Dementia-Rhetoric-to-Reality.pdf [Accessed 15 April 2021].

Phillipson, L. and Frost, D. (2020) 'Removing barriers to ethics approval: Innovation by a researcher and a person living with dementia', *The Australian Dementia Forum*, NHRMC National Institute for Dementia Research, E-Pub Abstract Booklet, p 47.

Swaffer, K. (2015) 'Dementia and Prescribed Disengagement™', *Dementia*, 14(1): 3–6.

13

Dementia, tourism and leisure: making the visitor economy dementia friendly

Joanne Connell and Stephen Page

Introduction

This chapter takes as its inspiration the well-established idea of living well with dementia and how this somewhat vague and contested idea might be effectively operationalised through an application to leisure and tourism businesses and activities. The purpose of this chapter is to give an overview of a nascent area of dementia-friendly activity: that of the visitor economy, which encompasses the range of businesses, services and spaces used by visitors to a neighbourhood, and often by local residents too. The interactions in, and value of, the largely neglected visitor economy concept within dementia studies is important as businesses and organisations that manage and promote place-based experiences and activities can enrich the lives of people with dementia, and their families and carers. This is relevant not only to visitors to a locale, but also to local residents, who also use and benefit from visitor economy businesses and services.

We review a programme of research that we have been pursuing to raise the profile of the visitor economy as an issue within both academic and practitioner agendas through tools and advocacy. Our principal focus throughout this research programme, which has involved different stakeholders (including those impacted by dementia in the community, and businesses and organisations that have responsibility for service delivery), is to enhance the accessibility of the visitor economy for people with dementia, thereby opening up neighbourhoods more fully so as to address a broader civil society objective of enhancing participation. This chapter also seeks to conceptualise these places as not just existing for residents, but also for visitors, and that people living with dementia exist in both categories. Our coverage in this chapter is necessarily selective but we seek to highlight some of the key dementia-related issues associated with the visitor economy and research and strategic responses that are starting to drive principles and practice forward. Our focus is on Great Britain although the principles we discuss have equal applicability within an international context.

Tourism and leisure as part of a dementia-friendly neighbourhood

Leisure as a broad concept encompasses a diverse spectrum of activity that incorporates long-haul travel through to going for a swim at a leisure centre and to home-based activities, such as knitting or watching television (see Page and Connell, 2010). Tourism, defined as travel away from the home for 24 hours or more, is a subset of leisure. Studies of the ageing population show that the nature, perception and scope of leisure changes through the life course and through generational cohorts. It is well established from time budget studies that those entering retirement have large proportions of their time available for leisure (see Gauthier and Smeeding, 2003). In this context, if a simple temporal view of leisure is adopted as the time available for pastimes and other non-work pursuits, the occurrence of diseases such as dementia creates a paradox in later life, where despite greater personal leisure time, opportunities to enjoy a range of activities, especially out of the home, may reduce. Classic studies of ageing and leisure identify that with increasing age comes decreasing leisure outside the home (see Nimrod and Janke, 2012) but studies such as Wearing (1995) and Bowling (2005) challenged dominant ideas about leisure engagement and involvement, particularly focusing on the more active ageing displayed by the baby boomer generation. In the 21st century, older people have become a distinctive, adventurous and lucrative tourist segment, recognised and cultivated by destination marketers and tourism corporations (Patterson, 2018).

But dementia is not framed by age alone, and the growing recognition of dementia as a disability opens up the field of accessible tourism where consideration is given to the ease of access of buildings, services and facilities are starting to become recognised. There is not only a moral imperative to facilitate access, but also a legal foundation. It is also recognised that disability does not prevent people from wanting to visit somewhere or be tourists, and likewise businesses recognise the value of developing their products and services for all markets. A significant body of knowledge and best practice on accessible tourism and leisure developed from the 1990s, but hidden conditions, including dementia and autism, have only recently been considered as part of mainstream inclusivity practices. For service businesses to cater for those with dementia within mainstream provision, a better understanding of the challenges that people with dementia face in their experiences and interactions with people, places and processes is needed, alongside understanding how adjustments that facilitate participation can make a significant difference. This resembles the discourse and actions around disability and accessibility that became more integrated into thinking in the visitor economy during the 1990s. In some countries, legislation is in place to ensure access to all and dementia is no exception to this (for example the Equality Act 2010 in the UK). Our two studies of England show that destination marketing organisations that specifically recognise dementia in their accessibility statements or web marketing are few and far between (Connell and Page, 2019a), while the number of businesses signed up as part of a dementia-friendly community[1] remains limited (Connell and Page, 2019b). We shall return to this work later in the chapter but first, the discussion turns to defining the scope of the visitor economy.

The visitor economy

The term visitor economy is not one widely used in the tourism, leisure and hospitality industries but one particularly favoured by the public sector to denote the amalgam of many parts that create value within a destination. As such, the term is designed to expand the breadth of the scope, scale and impact of those activities which fit within the tourism-leisure-hospitality-retailing domain that people engage with in their leisure time, and has significant resonance with the concept of neighbourhoods. As Tourism Toronto suggest 'the visitor economy – ... [is] ... a term much broader than tourism. Toronto's visitor economy encompasses the direct visitor spending in the destination and the indirect and induced economy activity that stems as a result' (Tourism Toronto 2019).

At an organisational level, the visitor economy incorporates the businesses, service providers and other groups engaged in providing, selling, marketing and/or facilitating the services used by visitors. It includes the broad tourism and hospitality sectors, such as accommodation, transport, visitor attractions, events, food and drink, cultural facilities, information services, tour guides and destination marketing organisations. The definition of a visitor is not simply a tourist, defined as on holiday and staying for at least one night away from home. Visitors are also people on day trips from home. Building a dementia-friendly visitor economy utilises facilities that overlap with other areas of dementia-friendly capacity building. Cafes, visitor attractions, bus services and museums are central to the visitor economy but also essential components of a dementia-friendly neighbourhood. In terms of both academic knowledge and business practice, Connell et al (2017) marked the first academic study of the degree of business engagement in the visitor economy with dementia as a growing societal issue. This study identified that a major challenge for the visitor economy is to meet the needs and expectations of a diverse public. From a mixed method study of visitor attractions in Scotland, several reasons for businesses' engagement with dementia were identified, including:

- for business development reasons, recognising the value of a new market segment;
- for personal or altruistic reasons and social responsibility goals;
- for regulatory and statutory reasons, requiring the design of measures to meet legislation to address disability inequalities and increase accessibility.

The focus on dementia and the visitor economy is increasingly important given the growing number of people affected by dementia, including those under the age of 65. Moreover, people with dementia do not necessarily conform to stereotypical images, and it is well established that living life to the full is valued by people with dementia, as it is for anyone. Organisations and businesses in the visitor economy have a distinct role to play in promoting quality of life and equality of provision so it is important that they are ready to welcome visitors with dementia and their carers (Connell and Page, 2019a).

Outings, day trips and holidays to tourist destinations (such as towns, cities, villages and seaside resorts), spaces (such as National Parks, the coast and countryside), sites (such as visitor attractions) and business premises (such as cafes and hotels) play an important role in quality of life for everyone in modern society. However, without an enabling framework that visibly promotes positive interactions between visitors, hosts and places, both the perception and lived experience of places can become a deterrent to visitors that live with dementia. Therein lies a significant challenge – how do we enable people with dementia to take advantage of leisure time to enhance well-being?

Living well with dementia: the role of tourism and leisure in a neighbourhood context

Proactive and positive approaches to the framing of dementia challenge the biomedical and socio-cultural constructions that tend to create disempowerment and retreat from the everyday in how society perceives dementia (Kontos, 2005). As Genoe (2010) argues in the case of dementia, leisure has the power to create a space where people can defy the stereotypes and stigma associated with the disease. These perspectives on what people *can* do, focus on the enabling and empowering facets of leisure, an idea that has become enshrined in policy and social consciousness, widely known as 'living well' with dementia. While the concept of living well has been criticised (for example Bartlett et al, 2017, p 178), it does help to place the idea of positivity and well-being at the heart of living with the condition, reducing the time-space compression that typifies social interaction, leisure experiences outside the home and the well-being impacts that these bring. This has become particularly important given the more recent shift towards earlier diagnoses, meaning that people may live with the early stages of the disease for some years. A second issue is that an increasing number of people are diagnosed at a younger age, and at a point in time where living life to the full is an accepted norm (Greenwood and Smith, 2016).

As Crampton et al (2012) argue, a diagnosis of dementia can result in withdrawal from leisure or recreational activities (including the places and sites which are frequented) because people with dementia may feel unwelcome or simply not recognised in the visitor economy. The prevailing policy view in England, popularised by the Prime Ministerial Challenge on Dementia (Department of Health, 2012), and which dominated health and social care practices in the community through the 2010s, focuses on understanding and providing the resources so that people can live as well as possible with dementia. This positive approach to operationalising the concept of personhood (Kitwood, 1997) and seeking non-clinical approaches to well-being with dementia, challenges conventional thinking on disability (Thomas and Milligan, 2015) and puts a focus on enabling and facilitating. How people live well with dementia is thought to be subject to a range of factors, and a recent study by Lamont et al (2020) emphasises the influence of psychological factors, including optimism and self-esteem. Activities that boost well-being and the psychological response to dementia, such as holidays and day trips, may thus contribute to living well. Given the wide range of types and symptoms of dementia, living with cognitive impairment brings progressive challenges that are experienced and countered by different people in different ways (Kitwood, 1997). The constraints imposed by dementia may be worked around with support, and holidays and days out may add to quality of life, boost family relationships and lessen negative feelings that might arise from the enclosing spatial prism associated with being at home. Watson (2016, p 5) argues that one aspect of living well with dementia is about 'having fun, in whatever form that takes' and the central issue here is that a diagnosis of dementia does not mean that seeking pleasure through activities like holidays and days out has to stop. Tourism and leisure can help to provide what Genoe and Dupuis (2014) term 'meaningful activity', which is so important for living well. Such meaningful activities are now commonly found in the community programmes within the arts and culture sector, particularly so in museums. Museums have spearheaded dementia-friendly initiatives in the visitor economy globally, for example in the US (Rhoads, 2009), New Zealand (McGuiggan et al, 2015), Spain (Belver et al, 2018) and many others. Museum experiences have been developed for and with people with dementia in the form of memory cafes, reminiscence sessions, art groups and object handling sessions, all of which are designed to promote memory, interaction, and personal and social interactions, emphasising the social role of museums (see Silverman, 2009). It is also very much the case that outdoor recreation may have a positive impact on emotional well-being (Duggan et al, 2008), for example in gardens (Whear et al, 2014; Liao, 2020), and woodlands (Cook, 2020). Being confined at home for long periods not only reduces opportunities for interaction with places and people that stimulate well-being, but may also escalate depression. Engaging in activities that a person and very often their carer-partner has always enjoyed can go some way to retaining a sense of normality (Roland and Chappell, 2015) and self-identity (Harman and Clare, 2006). Consequently, being able to continue doing pre-diagnosis activities can help to sustain feelings of well-being, maintain quality of life and even stave off accelerated deterioration, helping people to live at home for longer.

The desire to go on holiday or out for the day does not simply stop with the diagnosis of dementia (or even with symptoms but without a diagnosis). Prior to the onset of dementia, people are customers of a large number of businesses, shops and services. The need and motivation to use these services does not change after diagnosis or with the progression of dementia (Crampton et al, 2012). However, an individual's interaction with service providers will progressively change. Despite this commonsense observation, as Connell et al (2017) note, business engagement was not clearly understood or measured, with evidence of ad hoc rather than sector-wide initiatives and little attention in the academic literature until recent times. Crampton and Eley (2013) identify that if people cannot engage in everyday activities, there is a strong likelihood of withdrawing, which in turn impacts on well-being. As such, people with dementia need support in continuing with activities that have been a part of their life. Inherent in this is understanding dementia-friendly concepts from a supply side to encourage and enable businesses and services to adopt measures that can open up opportunities for everyone. To support the continued ability and confidence to use services and facilities, businesses and organisations working within the tourism and leisure sector, broadly labelled the visitor economy, need to be aware of the needs of a growing number of customers with dementia. Not only can greater awareness and action within the visitor economy benefit those travelling to enjoy visits to destinations for a holiday, a day out or to see family and friends, they can also contribute to the development of dementia-friendly communities for local residents.

In principle, tourism and leisure as a 'feel good activity' should contribute to living well and the positive view of 'doing things while you can' for people with mild to moderate dementia. We know from existing studies of dementia and leisure that outings and short journeys to local places and spaces make a significant contribution to living well through providing a boost to physical and mental well-being of people with dementia and their carers (see Page et al, 2015). That relationship is now much better understood than it was over a decade ago, and it is clear that local neighbourhoods offer myriad environments and experiences that contribute to well-being. Holidays and days out are an integral part of the modern social world (Page and Connell, 2020) but for people with dementia, the challenges of engaging in tourism and leisure present many barriers that may cause the individual's world to become more compressed in time and space. However, people with dementia and their carers strive to live well for as long as they can, and this includes going on holiday and day trips (Page et al, 2015; Innes et al, 2016). But this is not to underplay the reality of dementia in that taking part in once-enjoyed activities and experiences can be difficult physically, socially and emotionally. Bad experiences of going out for the day (such as insensitive or poor customer service, getting lost, unreliable public transport or not being able to locate a toilet) can be confusing, uncomfortable and frustrating and have the potential to stimulate negative feelings for people with dementia or can simply lead to avoidance and self-exclusion (Innes et al, 2016). One critical aspect is increasing the visibility of dementia as a condition that customers may present with. Tourism businesses are increasingly likely to come into contact with visitors with dementia and, as with other conditions and disabilities that are more visible, businesses need to become more aware of dementia and think about what they can do to make their service more inclusive. While dementia-friendly communities and support for local residents in accessing leisure facilities is improving, there is still some way to go to embed such principles in the wider visitor economy through the overt promotion of destinations (Connell and Page, 2019a). However, a neighbourhood approach to developing a more holistic recognition and welcoming of people within destinations and the businesses that comprise the visitor economy is important for several reasons. Not only can it mark out ways in which the visitor economy can serve the needs of a diverse public, but it can also consider ways in which a recognition of what works well for local residents works well for visitors. From a public policy or local government perspective, this approach encourages the joining up of multiple agendas in economic development, business support, tourism and community development. With some notable exceptions, few tourist destinations have adopted this approach and as we have found, links between dementia organisations (such as Dementia Action Alliances (DAAs) at the local level) and tourism destination marketing organisations are weak, if not non-existent, in many neighbourhood settings (Connell and Page, 2019a). Few destination marketing organisations (DMOs) belong to Dementia Friendly Communities or DAAs, and there is much potential to support the development of connections and initiatives that encompass the visitor economy as one strand of an innovative neighbourhood.

One of the key concepts we have used to explain how to expand access for people with dementia and their carers is touchpoints in the visitor journey. When people visit any place, defined as a destination, for a holiday or leisure undertaken in a timeframe where they return to their home at night, they will interact with different businesses, organisations and places that are called touchpoints during the visitor journey at the destination (Figure 13.1). This causes a degree of complexity in destinations where the number of elements that people interact with creates a significant challenge in progressing towards dementia readiness for destinations in ensuring each touchpoint is dementia friendly. One of the key challenges for any destination is to understand the nature of these touchpoints and where they take place. A further challenge is for one organisation to lead and coordinate the process and activities, with the input of people with dementia and their carers, and thus requires a strongly contextualised neighbourhood approach where people understand the places, spaces and services that it comprises. This is crucial for neighbourhoods and for the communities that seek to develop a dementia-friendly visitor economy, or even simply to support tourism businesses and organisations at an individual level. Furthermore, it is crucial to know where these touchpoints have the greatest significance for people with dementia and where the greatest opportunities and challenges exist (see Figure 13.1).

Touchpoints can of course occur before the site visit itself because getting to sites and venues is not without its problems, as Page et al (2015) and Innes et al (2016) found in terms of the transport and the travel experience. A lack of confidence about service encounters, social and environmental unfamiliarity, disorientation and a raft of accessibility issues can be a deterrent to experiencing the more positive benefits of taking a break or going out for the day, for both people with dementia and their carers.

Figure 13.1: Touchpoints in the visitor economy

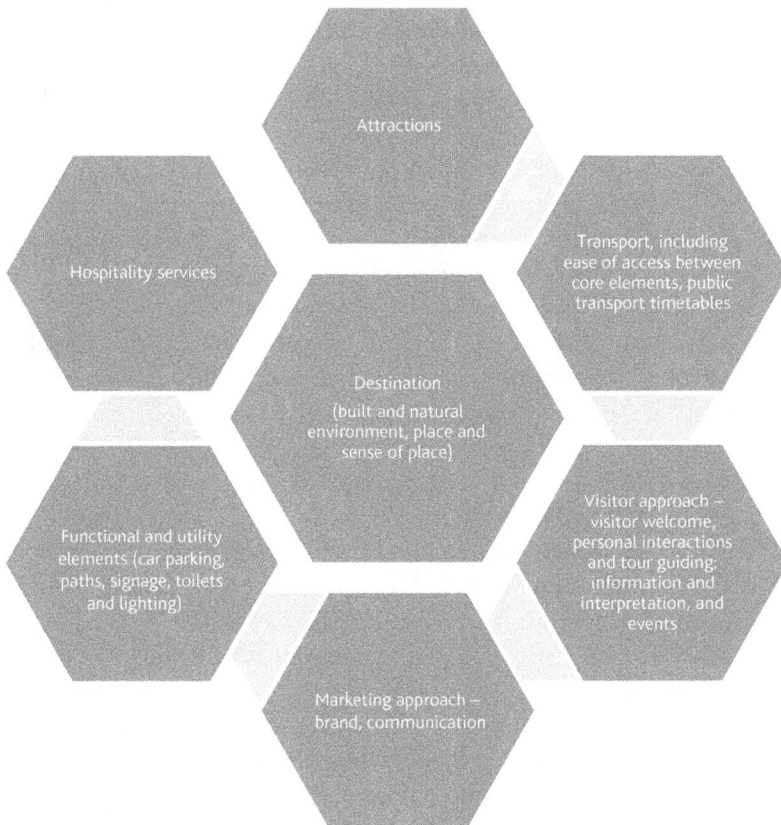

Source: Connell and Page (2019a, p 33)

Progress and best practice in the visitor economy

Our recent research, which has created a baseline of data, has focused on the nature and extent of dementia awareness in businesses and services within the visitor economy and sought to track and develop this to monitor emerging dementia friendliness in service provision. We have also worked with organisations to create guides for businesses and organisations that want to develop a more dementia-friendly approach to service provision. The discussion now turns to our major projects and the key findings, and influences on strategic thinking and policy for visitor organisations in the tourism and heritage sectors.

Business engagement study

The mixed method study by Connell et al (2017) set out (1) to assess dementia awareness in businesses; (2) identify skills, resource gaps and training needs for businesses seeking to become dementia friendly; (3) assess the extent of engagement in dementia-friendly initiatives; and (4) evaluate the experiences and perceptions of organisations in the visitor economy towards developing dementia-friendly leisure and tourism. Findings showed that businesses considered dementia to be an important issue but, with the exception of some leading advocates in the museums sector, it was yet to filter into actions. Further, there was some discomfort and reluctance around the topic, and there was no clear understanding of what 'dementia friendly' means. This perhaps raises the point of whether the term is simply too vague or whether more work needs to be done within subsectors of social and economic activity to promote broadly agreed principles. Where the term 'dementia friendly' is understood is clear: by those who have been affected by personal circumstances. For example, of those businesses already engaged in dementia-friendly initiatives, a personal, usually family, connection with dementia acted as the stimulus for action. Barriers to engagement included perceived costs of adaptations and concerns about knowledge and staff time, especially in small organisations. Dementia-friendly initiatives were found to be sporadic and non-uniform, indicating that facilitating advice and resources to help the visitor economy grow its dementia-ready capacity needed to be strengthened. In summary, the research showed that knowledge, resources, organisation and support are needed to build a dementia-friendly infrastructure. Businesses want to engage but do not always have the 'know how'. They need clear, tailored and targeted information on practical approaches if they are to adopt dementia-friendly approaches. Some of our early findings informed the creation of a toolkit for the National Coastal Tourism Academy (NCTA) Resource Hub. This is a web-based resource designed to provide advice to businesses operating in England's coastal areas on how to adopt a range of dementia-friendly actions (https://coastaltourismacademy.co.uk/resource-hub/resource/dementia-why-is-it-important-for-tourism).

Guidance for the heritage sector

Given the broad scope of the visitor economy, and the overlap with community resources, there are many opportunities to create and further develop dementia-friendly approaches for service visitors and local residents alike. One sector that has been highlighted as particularly appealing for people with dementia and their carers is the heritage sector, and in particular historic houses and gardens. Through interviews with people with dementia and their carers, Innes et al (2016) identified that heritage sites are perceived as a 'safe' and relaxed environment with the right type of services on offer, such as toilets and a cafe. The characteristics of many heritage sites make them particularly suitable for visits by care home groups as well as independent visits. Many heritage sites exhibit the key attributes that visitors with dementia and their carers seek, such as safe outdoor environments with space to walk, wander or use wheelchairs, a relaxed and uncrowded environment, and clear signage, entrance and exit points. In addition, the social interaction with staff and volunteers gives the feeling of being looked after.

Work to make the heritage sector more dementia friendly has been advocated by a group of heritage site managers led by Historic Royal Palaces in the guise of the Dementia-Friendly Heritage Network. Historic Royal Palaces led an initiative to create a guide for heritage site managers designed to communicate ways to make sites more welcoming and accessible to people with dementia and their carers. This guide, *Rethinking Heritage: A Guide to Help Make Your Site More Dementia-Friendly* (Klug et al, 2017) has been widely circulated within the heritage sector and is being used at heritage sites across the country. Evaluation shows that levels of awareness of dementia and ways in which sites could be adapted after reading the Guide increased. Guide users were definitively able to evidence changes and adaptations to their existing practices as a result of increased awareness after reading the Guide. The user orientation of the Guide made its content and knowledge easily transferable, through top tips and case studies. A wide range of new activities undertaken after reading the Guide were listed by users and the identification of how to overcome obstacles to implementing new practices was noted as a strength of the Guide. Users identified the remaining barriers to becoming more dementia friendly as primarily related to the structural nature of the site in that the protected nature of ancient buildings meant that physical adaptations were very difficult. Furthermore, the future availability of funding sources to finance new promotions, more costly environmental design changes or adaptations for initiatives was viewed as an issue in moving forward. Despite this, the Heritage Guide was cited by a National Trust (2019) press release on its evolving relationship with the Alzheimer's Society in making its 500 sites dementia friendly, which highlights the special connection between historic sites and benefits for people with dementia:

> historic spaces, collections and stories can prompt and stimulate discussion and connection, encourage outdoor exploration, and offer a vital connection to the world around them, with day trips recognised as one of the most likely and regular activities for people living with the condition and their carers (National Trust, 2019).

National guide for tourism businesses

One of the findings of Connell et al (2017) was that businesses had little 'know how' in making some progress towards becoming dementia friendly. The national tourism organisations Visit England and Visit Scotland produced a guide *Dementia-friendly Tourism: A Practical Guide for Businesses* (2019), to which we contributed through the working group. This guide tackles the issue of 'know how' head on by setting out easy steps that all businesses can take and providing supportive advice. The preparation of this guide was based on a collaborative process, including people with dementia and their experiences of going to attractions and staying in holiday accommodation, alongside businesses that had already taken some steps to more effectively welcome people with dementia. This guide, aimed primarily at small to medium sized enterprises (SMEs) in the accommodation sector and visitor attractions, outlined a series of simple, low-cost, practical ideas that businesses could introduce. The guide identified the reasons for businesses to become more dementia friendly and presented three key themes: *information* (for example promoting dementia-friendly services and providing information for people with dementia beforehand so informed decisions can be made about planning a visit); *people* (for example staff awareness and training, or understanding how to communicate well); and *place* (for example making physical adaptations and providing clear signage).

Future prospects

Given the health-promoting effects on physical and mental well-being, finding ways to support people living with dementia to enjoy time away from home is vital in the development and recognition of dementia-friendly approaches to people, place and business contexts if one builds on the Crampton et al (2012, 2013) studies. But it is not sufficient to simply recognise that holidays and days out are good for people as a break from the norm or a chance to refresh and rejuvenate given the scale and diversity of the visitor economy. If one starts from the premise that the visitor economy can engage more fully to reduce the barriers from a supply-side perspective, what are the existing barriers to businesses? Understanding and awareness of dementia within the visitor economy is developing through the initiatives outlined in this chapter, although there is still some way to go to embed these principles into mainstream practice (Connell and Page, 2019a, 2019b). Recent experience in working on guides for service settings (Klug et al, 2017; Visit England et al, 2019) demonstrates that a wide range of stakeholders need to be engaged in designing and developing the case study material as well as the differing motives and agendas which these stakeholders have. This is a far from easy process when bringing together academics, NGOs, large charities, QUANGOS, and people with dementia and their carers in an attempt to reach out in a user-friendly way to business owners and managers. Reaching and communicating with a wide range of stakeholders to provide world-leading and innovative materials is critical, as the example of the Visit England and Visit Scotland (2019) *Dementia-Friendly Tourism Guide* shows: within three months of its initial online launch, 31 organisations had embraced it within their own organisational work or disseminated it to a much wider global audience in countries such as China and across Asia. What we hope to have shown in this snapshot of our work is what the UK Department for Business, Innovation and Skills (2010) *Science for All* report summarised as the process of public engagement as three interconnected points on a triangle comprising: *Collaboration* (for example through co-created research and consensus building with public audiences); *Transmission* (for example communicating knowledge to diverse audiences through press releases, public relations campaigns, podcasts and social media);

and *Receiving* (for example collecting feedback, input to the research process by the public through surveys, consultations and interviews). We are still working actively on the latter aspects of that listening and receiving function as we seek to synthesise feedback in helping to develop and contribute to the design of more dementia-friendly visitor experiences that we hope will gradually be shared globally. Our work also raises a number of moral issues, specifically when looking at spaces which are consumed for leisure and tourism: Who are these spaces for? Who has the right to be in these places and what actions do we need to take to ensure that these are accessible for all? This is informed by a long tradition of research, emanating from studies such as Lefebvre's *Rights to the City* (Lefebvre, 1973) which transcend many of the current legal-compliance debates around equality acts in many countries to ensure people, irrespective of their personal situation, have a right to access spaces and places for whatever reason.

In conclusion, the visitor economy might be viewed by some as an insignificant, tangential or at best supplementary aspect of a neighbourhood approach to dementia. However, the visitor economy is slowly being recognised as part of a neighbourhood approach to progressing dementia-friendly attributes. The benefits of tourism and leisure to people living within the locale in the form of places to go are clear but the added aspect of developing a dementia-friendly neighbourhood that is attractive to visitors is a relatively new area of inquiry and strategic interest. Holidays and outings are important to subjective quality of life and may also have a role to play in physical well-being through exercise and gaining the benefits of the outdoors. The chapter has shown the emerging recognition and interest of a range of service providers in the visitor economy but not knowing how to address dementia within service operations has been an inhibitor to development. Understanding the touchpoints in the visitor journey are crucial, and while these are different in each service setting, there are broad similarities that can be assessed and acted on using support available through new sector-specific guidance. Organisations in the heritage and tourism sectors are working to stimulate action by leading by example and demonstrating simple steps that can make a difference. However, in a context where business priorities are stretched, particularly post pandemic, further progress remains a challenge.

Note

[1] We use the term community in this context as much of the literature and initiatives around becoming dementia-friendly emanate in the UK from the Alzheimer's Society's pursuit of creating dementia-friendly communities. These communities can

exist at a variety of spatial scales from the city or village to a local neighbourhood and so for consistency we use the term neighbourhood rather than community as the two are synonymous if approaching this issue from the perspective of lead organisations that have promoted place-based approaches to becoming dementia friendly initially that then incorporated business types (see Connell and Page, 2019b for a more detailed discussion of the evolution of this strand of becoming a dementia-friendly community).

References

Bartlett, R., Windemuth-Wolfson, L., Oliver, K. and Dening, T. (2017) 'Suffering with dementia: The other side of "living well"', *International Psychogeriatrics*, 29(2): 177–9.

Belver, M., Ullán, A., Avila, N., Moreno, C. and Hernández, C. (2018) 'Art museums as a source of well-being for people with dementia: An experience in the Prado Museum', *Arts & Health*, 10(3): 213–26.

Bowling, A. (2005) *Ageing Well: Quality of Life in Old Age*, Maidenhead: Open University Press.

Connell, J. and Page, S.J. (2019a) 'Destination-readiness for dementia-friendly visitor experiences: A scoping study', *Tourism Management*, 70: 9–41.

Connell, J. and Page, S.J. (2019b) 'An exploratory study of creating dementia-friendly businesses in the visitor economy: Evidence from the UK', *Heliyon*, 5(4): e01471.

Connell, J., Page, S.J., Sherriff, I. and Hibbert, J. (2017) 'Business engagement in a civil society: Transitioning towards a dementia-friendly visitor economy', *Tourism Management*, 61: 110–28.

Cook, M. (2020) 'Using urban woodlands and forests as places for improving the mental well-being of people with dementia', *Leisure Studies*, 39(1): 41–55.

Crampton, J., Dean, J. and Eley, R. (2012) *Creating a Dementia-Friendly York*. York: Joseph Rowntree Foundation.

Crampton, J. and Eley, R. (2013) 'Dementia-friendly communities: What the project "Creating a dementia-friendly York" can tell us', *Working with Older People*, 17(2): 49–57.

Department of Health (2012) *Prime Minister's Challenge on Dementia: Delivering major improvements in dementia care and research by 2015*, London: DoH.

Duggan, S., Blackman, T., Martyr, A. and Van Schaike, P. (2008) 'The impact of early dementia on an outdoor life: A shrinking world?' *Dementia: The International Journal of Social Research and Practice*, 7(2): 191–204.

Gauthier, A. and Smeeding, T. (2003) 'Time use at older ages: Cross-national differences', *Research on Aging*, 25(3): 247–74.

Genoe, R.M. (2010) 'Leisure as resistance within the context of dementia', *Leisure Studies*, 29(3): 303–20.

Genoe, R.M. and Dupuis, S.L. (2014) 'The role of leisure within the dementia context', *Dementia*, 13(1): 33–58.

Greenwood, N. and Smith, R. (2016) 'The experiences of people with young–onset dementia: A meta–ethnographic review of the qualitative literature', *Maturitas*, 92: 102–9.

Harman, G. and Clare, L. (2006) 'Illness representations and lived experience in early-stage dementia', *Qualitative Health Research*, 16(4): 484–502.

Innes, A., Page, S.J. and Cutler, C. (2016) 'Barriers to leisure participation for people with dementia and their carers: An exploratory analysis of carer and people with dementia's experiences', *Dementia*, 15(6): 1643–65.

Kitwood, T. (1997) *Dementia reconsidered: The person comes first*. Milton Keynes: Open University Press.

Klug, K., Page, S.J., Connell, J., Robson, D. and Bould, E. (2017) *Rethinking Heritage: A Guide to Help Make Your Site More Dementia-Friendly*, London: Historic Royal Palaces.

Kontos, P.C. (2005) 'Embodied selfhood in Alzheimer's disease: Rethinking person-centred care', *Dementia*, 4(4): 553–70.

Lamont, R., Nelis, S., Quinn, C., Martyr, A., Rippon, I., Kopelman, M., Hindle, J., Jones, R., Litherland, R. and Clare, L. (2020) 'Psychological predictors of "living well" with dementia: Findings from the IDEAL study', *Aging & Mental Health*, 24(6): 956–64.

Lefebvre, H. (1973) *La survie du capitalisme; la re-production des rapports de production*, trans Frank Bryant as *The Survival of Capitalism*, London: Allison and Busby, 1976.

Liao, M-L., Ou, S-J., Heng Hsieh, C., Li, Z. and Ko, C-C. (2020) 'Effects of garden visits on people with dementia: A pilot study', *Dementia*, 19(4): 1009–28.

National Trust (2019) 'Two of the UK's most popular charities have today announced an ambitious three-year project to unlock some of the nation's best loved history and heritage for millions of people affected by dementia', available from: https://www. nationaltrust.org.uk/press-release/unlocking-history-and-heritage-for-millions-of-people-affected-by-dementia#:~:text=The%20 National%20Trust%20is%20joining,its%20kind%20for%20the%20 Trust.&text=In%20comparison%20to%20other%20visitor,'safe'%20 and%20familiar%20spaces [Accessed 15 April 2021].

Nimrod, G. and Janke, M. (2012) 'Leisure across the later life span', in Gibson, H. and Singleton, J. (eds) *Leisure and Aging: Theory and Practice*, Champaign: Human Kinetics, pp 95–110.

Page, S. and Connell, J. (2010) *Leisure: An Introduction*, Harlow: Pearson Education Limited.

Page, S.J. and Connell, J. (eds) (2020) *The Routledge Handbook of Events*, Abingon: Routledge.

Page, S.J., Innes, A. and Cutler, C. (2015) 'Developing dementia-friendly tourism destinations: An exploratory analysis', *Journal of Travel Research*, 54(4): 467–81.

Patterson, I. (2018) *Tourism and Leisure Behaviour in an Ageing World*, Wallingford: CABI.

Rhoads, L. (2009) 'Museums, meaning making, and memories: The need for museum programs for people with dementia and their caregivers', *Curator: The Museum Journal*, 52(3): 229–40.

Roland, K.P. and Chappell, N.L. (2015) 'Meaningful activity for persons with dementia: Family caregiver perspectives', *American Journal of Alzheimer's Disease & Other Dementias*, September: 559–68

Silverman, L. (2009) *The Social Work of Museums*, Abingdon: Routledge.

Thomas, C. and Milligan, C. (2015) *How Can and Should UK Society Adjust to Dementia?* York: Joseph Rowntree Foundation Viewpoint Paper.

Tourism Toronto (2019) Toronto's visitor economy: an economic catalyst for the city and the region, Toronto: Tourism Toronto, https://partners.seetorontonow.com/wp-content/uploads/sites/7/2019/11/Toronto-Visitor-Economy-final.pdf [Accessed 28 April 2021].

UK Department for Business, Innovation and Skills (2010) *Science for All*, London: UK Department for Business, Innovation and Skills.

Visit England (2019) Dementia friendly tourism: a practical guide for businesses. https://www.visitbritain.org/sites/default/files/vb-corporate/business-hub/resources/dementia_friendly_guide_for_tourism_businesses.pdf [Accessed 28 April 2021].

Watson, J. (2016) 'Is it possible to live well with dementia?', *Dementia*, 15(1): 4–5.

Wearing, B. (1995) 'Leisure and resistance in an ageing society', *Leisure Studies*, 14(4): 263–79.

Whear, R., Thompson Coon, J., Bethel, A., Abbott, R., Stein, K. and Garside, R. (2014) 'What is the impact of using outdoor spaces such as gardens on the physical and mental well-being of those with dementia? A systematic review of quantitative and qualitative evidence', *Journal of the American Medical Directors Association*, 15(10): 697–705.

14

Conclusion: Dementia emplaced

Andrew Clark, Richard Ward and Lyn Phillipson

Thinking through dementia and place

In the Introduction to this book, we proposed that dementia and place are co-constitutive, discursively and experientially, but to date this relationship has yet to be given full consideration. This is not to overlook an extensive tradition of research into dementia and the environment, but rather to suggest that an explicit focus on how dementia comes to shape understandings and experiences of place, and vice versa, remains underdeveloped in the field of dementia studies. The preceding chapters find common ground or, more accurately, share a common starting point, of seeking to understand experiences of dementia through the locational lens of the neighbourhood. Yet while most of the chapters start out from here, few end up at the same end point. In part, this may be because a *neighbourhood* is a somewhat slippery concept, implying simultaneously a scale of perspective as well as a lived phenomenon worth investigating. Indeed, what emerges overall is how neighbourhoods can offer a particular position from which to enhance our understanding of life with dementia and, in turn, of how living with dementia provides sometimes unique and valuable ways of knowing what neighbourhoods are about.

The chapters demonstrate the diversity of theoretical and conceptual thinking about how we might approach and understand place-based experiences for those living with dementia. They also inform and extend the conceptual and theoretical stock of dementia studies, drawing on ideas already in circulation, such as personhood and social citizenship (Chapter 10), and borrowing from other disciplines and perspectives, such as transactional perspectives and place integration (Chapter 4), relational space (Chapter 2), models of social health (Chapter 11) and performativity (Chapter 7). The need for renewed attention to conceptual thinking about people in 'local' environments is explicitly seen in Seetharaman and colleagues' (Chapter 8) exploration of the dynamic relationship between the person living with dementia and neighbourhood environments, which seeks to better integrate the physical and psychosocial dimensions of the neighbourhood environment in people's lives. The result there, and indeed across the book, are attempts to think differently not so much about life with dementia, but about life with dementia in and through place.

If we accept that neighbourhoods are socially produced (Lefebvre, 1991), then this book provides some cautious optimism about how to create more equal and fairer places for those living with dementia. This productive capacity has been presented at a practical as well as conceptual level. For instance, as Connell and Page (Chapter 13) demonstrate, developing the visitor economy can bring the benefits of tourism and leisure to local residents as well as visitors in ways that have seldom been considered in the dementia-friendly movement, while Ward and colleagues (Chapter 7) point to the ways in which dementia activism and advocacy can contribute to the creation of more equal experiences of neighbourhood life for all. As the chapters by Phinney et al (Chapter 10) and Ward et al (Chapter 7) also show, recognising the opportunities and capacities for self-advocacy, as well as the broader agency of people living with dementia, is one way of overcoming pathologising and deterministic approaches to dementia in place.

Many of the chapters in this book place the experiences of those living with dementia and care partners centre stage (see Chapter 3, Chapter 6, Chapter 9, Chapter 12). For instance, Odzakovic and colleagues (Chapter 5) show that people living alone with dementia can, and do, actively engage in planned and spontaneous initiatives and interactions to remain connected. But such activity is itself relational, and at times starkly dependent on, the support of other individuals as well as services and a broader neighbourhood infrastructure (see also Chapter 8 and Chapter 13).

While we already know something of how neighbourhoods as social locations might change over time for those living with dementia (Duggan et al, 2008; Ward et al, 2018), we hope that this book makes a further contribution to understanding how people living with dementia really engage with changes in and to localities. Public and outdoor settings are complex, challenging and potentially exclusionary, be that in terms of accessibility and navigation (Chapter 4), socially (Chapter 5) or economically (Chapter 13). As Brennan-Horley and colleagues (Chapter 11) explore, we must continue to recognise and address this complexity without recourse to pathologising discourses of place that construct environments outside of the home as risky and feared. Rather than simply dismissing such risks and fears, this book offers a more nuanced set of accounts of neighbourhoods as places of possibility – without homogenising that experience. It remains vital to avoid the reductivism of a single 'neighbourhood experience' for those living with dementia or by dichotomising places as either 'dementia friendly' or not (Chapter 2, Chapter 11). Hence, while neighbourhoods can provide webs of (social) support and facilitate engagement and activism, we should not romanticise this potential (Chapter 2, Chapter 3, Chapter 7). Those who live alone, for instance, have rather different experiences (Chapter 5) and there is a need to recognise and work within local contexts to understand how global as well as local politics, economies and cultures intersect with social, civic and material properties. The chapters demonstrate the ongoing importance of space and place as mediators of well-being, sociability, citizenship and engagement in the everyday lives of people with dementia. In proposing such a shift from thinking of places like neighbourhoods as some*where* we inhabit to some*thing* we do, we hope that this book has offered some ideas and indicators of where this alternative conception might lead.

Limitations and omissions

This is certainly not the final word on attempts to understand dementia and place. Inevitably, our decision to encourage contributors to start from the site and scale of local experience means that we have barely touched on the myriad of different places that matter when it comes to understanding life with dementia. So here we consider potential limitations to a neighbourhoods lens for understanding the emplaced lives of people with dementia. We also highlight broader patterns in dementia studies, where certain experiences of place have consistently been given prominence over others, and the need for research to redress this.

The idea of a neighbourhood implies an urban bias that holds particular meaning within the Global North, especially for nations across Europe, North America and Australasia. It forms part of a self-referential discourse on place within minority affluent countries that has consistently failed to address place-based experiences and approaches to dementia in the Global South. Yet, we would argue for using 'neighbourhood' as an heuristic; a banner under which to explore the relationship between people and places, with potentially international and cross-cultural applicability. Ultimately though, perhaps the term 'neighbourhood' is less relevant than the more widely shared experiences that it draws together: questions of proximity, reciprocity, sociality and belonging. Clearly, there is a need for further research into the experience of local living for people with dementia across different cultural and geographic contexts. As organisations such as the World Health Organization and Alzheimer's Disease International promote a Dementia Friendly Communities agenda on a global scale (ADI, 2017; WHO, 2018) it is imperative that such initiatives actively consider, and build upon, situated knowledge and understanding of people's relationship to place when living with dementia to avoid the risk of cultural imperialism.

Not unrelated is the question of what role place and neighbourhoods play in the lives of migrant groups and communities affected by dementia. There is a small but growing cluster of research into transnational perspectives on dementia that highlights the complexities of people's relationship to place over time. Past experiences are carried forward, often in embodied forms, and used to transform neighbourhood spaces through importing social practices and relations and ways of conducting local life. To date, much existing commentary tends to foreground the experience of caregivers or is offered from the caregiver's perspective (Brijnath, 2009; Naess et al, 2015; Parmar and Puwar, 2019; Chaouni et al, 2020). Much could be learned from exploring the experience of neighbourhood living for migrants with dementia, to understand how people find ways to anchor themselves in the present while holding on to familiar aspects of the past.

The urban-centric orientation of some approaches to neighbourhoods may underplay rural experiences of dementia and of living in geographically remote locations, both of which remain under-researched in the field of dementia studies (Innes et al, 2020). There are particular challenges and considerations in the design and implementation of support services in rural settings (Bowes et al, 2018; Innes et al, 2020). Yet much existing research focuses upon caregivers rather than the perspective and experience of the person with dementia (Sun et al, 2010; Innes et al, 2011; Orpin et al, 2014; Herron et al, 2019). Blackstock and colleagues (2006) caution against binary thinking towards rural and urban conditions in a dementia context and reveal the diverse experience of rurality for people living with dementia and are critical of a 'generalising narrative of the rural idyll' in how people's experience is represented and interpreted. We might add that a similar caution needs to be applied when thinking about urban and suburban locations.

Indeed, Keady et al (2012) identified a similar problem in much of the earlier research on dementia and neighbourhoods. The authors point to the use of generalising references to 'the outdoors', 'the built environment' and 'public space' rather than more specific accounts of particular places at certain points in time, and a consequent failure to acknowledge the socio-economic variations that differentiate neighbourhood experiences for people with dementia. Our argument for a 'neighbourhood-centred' approach is aimed at problematising these representational and generic notions of place embedded in much existing policy, in favour of research that deals more directly with the lived experience of neighbourhood (see also Ward et al, 2018). Writing in the related field of critical disability studies, Goodley and colleagues (2019) have highlighted the failure of much published research to situate itself and consequently encourage disability scholars to be clear, open and honest about their own local locations, 'rather than assuming the reader knows all about say, the British context' (p 979). This is an argument for the situating of research, as well as collective understandings of a condition such as dementia, in the contexts in which it is produced, and to be aware of the limits of that understanding.

There is growing recognition of the importance of attention to the diversity of people affected by dementia, including underrepresented groups such as ethnic minorities (for example Botsford et al, 2012), LGBT+ groups (for example Westwood and Price, 2016), people with young onset dementia (for example Greenwood and Smith, 2016), people with dementia who live alone (for example Chapter 5), and people with intellectual disabilities (for example Watchman, 2017). Hulko (2009) uses intersectionality to frame the ongoing interactions of different forms of oppression experienced by individuals living with dementia, arguing that policy and practice must attend to the widely differing experience of dementia based on a person's social situation. Yet, existing research into the experience of dementia for communities of identity tends to overlook space and place and ignores the emplaced experiences of people with dementia. A focus on place may help to inform an intersectional understanding of dementia, through an appreciation of how place is implicated in the open-ended and processual nature of identity. For instance, a case study offered by O'Connor and colleagues (2010) highlights how an alternative cultural understanding of place for a First Nation Canadian woman shapes her experience of living with dementia.

Crucially though, silences remain about the lived experience of place for people living with dementia (McGovern, 2017; Calvert et al, 2020). Though of value, much research remains clustered around policy and providers' concerns for service provision, support mechanisms and the efficacy of 'community-based' interventions. Yet the very notion of a dementia-friendly community implies the involvement of a broader range of neighbourhood players and places in the lives of people with dementia. Far greater emphasis needs to be given to this wider network of relationships and the priorities expressed by people with dementia themselves regarding the everyday challenges of living with dementia in a neighbourhood setting.

A beginning not an ending

We hope this book will provide an opening to a more critical debate on dementia and place, providing food for thought both for policy ambitions for the emerging Dementia Friendly Communities agenda and efforts to more knowingly incorporate place within dementia care practice. We end by highlighting messages from the collected chapters to guide future directions for policy, research and practice.

Policy

Existing place-based policy on dementia has begun to coalesce around the notion of dementia-friendly communities. The idea borrows heavily from the more established Age Friendly Cities and Communities (AFCC) movement and until now has left unchecked the assumption that what works for ageing and later life will necessarily work for people with dementia. While recognising the potential for learning and dialogue with AFCC initiatives, this book sounds a note of caution on three counts. First, policy makers may benefit from looking beyond standard responses for locational domains to consider the 'particularities of place' (Handler, 2019) in the lives of people with dementia (Chapter 4, Chapter 7). Second, in doing this, questions need to be asked about how place itself is understood and approached in dementia policy (Chapter 2, Chapter 11). And third, by thinking more critically about place, policy makers should revisit assumptions about how to influence positive change at a neighbourhood level and the impact of that change upon the lives of people with dementia (Chapter 5, Chapter 7).

Research

While it is clear that the dementia-friendly agenda is an applied and 'hands-on' movement for change in which research has a role to play, this book highlights the importance of a critical and theorised framing of this agenda. Thus, while it is crucial to collaborate with people living with dementia to understand the approaches to neighbourhood change that are most effective and beneficial, the research community should also ensure close links with theoretical developments to avoid fossilised thinking (Chapter 8). As Brennan-Horley and colleagues (Chapter 11) have shown, research can innovate through experimental and exploratory methods for engaging and empowering people living with dementia to influence the production of place, while Connell and Page (Chapter 13) have demonstrated how research has a role to play in questioning the silences and gaps in organisational and industry-wide practice pertaining to dementia and place. While we believe that the neighbourhood lens can make a significant contribution to critical dementia studies, further contributions will benefit from interdisciplinary thinking while embracing ideas new to the field. This includes emergent thinking around non-representational theory (for example Jeong, 2020), new materialism (for example Buse and Twigg, 2016; Ren and Strickfaden, 2018) and post-humanist perspectives (for example Quinn and Blandon, 2017; Jenkins et al, 2020). While we are not advocating the uncritical integration of such, they do have much potential to provide fresh insight into place-based perspectives on the lived experience of dementia.

Practice

Implications for practice are manifold but centre upon the core message that place matters for managing life with dementia. The chapters in this book demonstrate that dementia practice is no longer exclusively the domain of health and social care (Chapter 13). Planners, architects, engineers, retailers, business leaders, workers in sports and leisure, arts and culture and those in the service sector are all now implicated in connection with people with dementia (Chapter 10). Looking ahead, we need to better recognise the diversification of practice and how best to enlist this more widely (and thinly) distributed support at both local and national levels. In their chapter on people living alone with dementia, Odzakovic and colleagues (Chapter 5) warn of the danger of creating 'normative neighbourhoods' through place-based initiatives that fail to acknowledge the diversity of people living with dementia. Arguably, the heterogeneity of those with dementia poses one of the greatest challenges for services and support. Indeed, some commentators on the age-friendly cities agenda have questioned whether it is even realistic to try and assist a broad cross-section of older people (Golant, 2014) in the context of finite resources. In this respect practitioners have a role to play in empowering people with dementia to hold policy makers to account (Chapter 11) and in ensuring that community development initiatives are responsive to the diversity of people living with dementia (Chapter 9, Chapter 12).

Ultimately, this book has only been possible as a result of the individual and collective contributions of people living with dementia and their care partners. The narratives and experiences gathered here demonstrate that places such as neighbourhoods are more than a useful resource but a place of belonging, connection, friendship and love (Chapter 3, Chapter 6, Chapter 9, Chapter 12). Perhaps, then, the most important message in this book concerns the individual and collective potential of people with dementia, and those who support them, to not only change the course of their own journeys with the condition, but also through their actions to contribute to fairer and more equitable places for us all to live.

References

Alzheimer's Disease International (2017) *Dementia Friendly Communities: Global developments*, 2nd edn [online], available from: https://www.alzheimers.org.nz/getattachment/News-and-Events/Global-information/Alzheimer-s-Disease-International-Report/Alzheimers-Disease-International-2.pdf/ [Accessed 05 February 2021].

Blackstock, K.L., Innes, A., Cox, S. Smith, A. and Mason, A. (2006) 'Living with dementia in rural and remote Scotland: Diverse experiences of people with dementia and their carers', *Journal of Rural Studies*, 22(2): 161–76.

Botsford, J., Clarke C.L. and Gibb C.E. (2012) 'Dementia and relationships: Experiences of partners in minority ethnic communities', *Journal of Advanced Nursing*, 68(10): 2207–17.

Bowes, A., Dawson, A. and McCabe, L. (2018) 'RemoDem: Delivering support for people with dementia in remote areas', *Dementia*, 17(3): 297–314.

Brijnath, B. (2009) 'Familial bonds and boarding passes: Understanding caregiving in a transnational context', *Identities*, 16(1): 83–101.

Buse, C. and Twigg, J. (2016) 'Materialising memories: Exploring the stories of people with dementia through dress', *Ageing and Society*, 36(6): 1115–35.

Calvert, L., Keady, J., Khetani, B., Riley, C. and Swarbrick, C. (2020) '"This is my home and my neighbourhood with my very good and not so good memories": The story of autobiographical place-making and a recent life with dementia', *Dementia*, 19: 111–28.

Chaouni, S.B., Smetcoren, A.-S. and de Donder, L. (2020) 'Caring for migrant older Moroccans with dementia in Belgium as a complex and dynamic transnational network of informal and professional care: A qualitative study', *International Journal of Nursing Studies*, 101: 103415.

Duggan, S., Blackman, T., Martyr, A. and Van Schaike, P. (2008) 'The impact of early dementia on an outdoor life: A shrinking world?' *Dementia*, 7(2): 191–204.

Golant, S.M. (2014) 'Age-friendly communities: Are we expecting too much?' *IRPP Insight*, 2(5): 1–19.

Goodley, D., Lawthom, R., Liddiard K. and Runswick-Cole, K. (2019) 'Provocations for Critical Disability Studies', *Disability & Society*, 34(6): 972–97.

Greenwood, N. and Smith, R. (2016) 'The experiences of people with young-onset dementia: A meta-ethnographic review of the qualitative literature', *Maturitas*, 92: 102–9.

Handler, S. (2019) 'Alternative age-friendly initiatives: Redefining age-friendly design', in Buffel, T., Handler, S. and Phillipson, C. (eds) *Age-friendly Cities and Communities: A Global Perspective*, Bristol: Policy Press.

Herron, R. and Rosenberg, M. (2019) 'Dementia in rural settings: Examining the experiences of former partners in care', *Ageing and Society*, 39(2): 340–57.

Hulko, W. (2009) 'From "not a big deal" to "hellish": Experiences of older people with dementia', *Journal of Aging Studies*, 23(3): 131–44.

Innes, A., Morgan, D. and Farmer, J. (2020) *Remote and Rural Dementia Care: Policy, Research and Practice*, Bristol: Policy Press.

Innes, A., Morgan, D. and Kosteniuk, J. (2011) 'Dementia care in rural and remote settings: A systematic review of informal/family caregiving', *Maturitas*, 68(1): 34–46.

Jenkins, N., Ritchie, L. and Quinn, S. (2020) 'From reflection to diffraction: Exploring the use of vignettes within posthumanist and multi-species research', *Qualitative Research*, 1–25. Online Firstview, available from: https://journals.sagepub.com/doi/pdf/10.1177/1468794120920258 [Accessed 28 April 2021].

Jeong, J.M. (2020) 'The affective creativity of a couple in dementia care', *Culture, Medicine and Psychiatry*, 44: 360–81.

Keady, J., Campbell, S., Barnes, H., Ward, R., Li, X., Swarbrick, C., Burrow, S. and Elvish, R. (2012) 'Neighbourhoods and dementia in the health and social care context: A realist review of the literature and implications for UK policy development', *Reviews in Clinical Gerontology*, 22(2): 150–63.

Lefebvre, H. (1991) *The Production of Space*, trans D. Nicholson-Smith, Oxford: Wiley.

McGovern, J. (2017) 'Capturing the significance of place in the lived experience of dementia', *Qualitative Social Work*, 16(5): 664–79.

O'Connor, D., Phinney, A. and Hulko, W. (2010) 'Dementia at the intersections: A unique case study exploring social location', *Journal of Aging Studies*, 24(1): 30–9.

Orpin, P., Stirling, C., Hetherington, S. and Robinson, A. (2014) 'Rural dementia carers: Formal and informal sources of support', *Ageing and Society*, 34(2): 185–208.

Parmar, P. and Puwar, N. (2019) 'Striking a chord', *Performance Research*, 24(1): 25–34.

Quinn, J. and Blandon, C. (2017) 'The potential for lifelong learning in dementia: A post-humanist exploration', *International Journal of Lifelong Education*, 36(5): 578–94.

Ren, H. and Strickfaden, M. (2018) 'The active role of material things: An environment-based conceptual framework to understand the well-being of people with dementia', *Open Journal of Social Sciences*, 6: 11–23.

Sun, F., Kosberg, J.I., Kaufman A.V. and Leeper, J.D. (2010) 'Coping strategies and caregiving outcomes among rural dementia caregivers', *Journal of Gerontological Social Work*, 53(6): 547–67.

Ward, R., Clark, A., Campbell, S., Graham, B., Kullberg, A., Manji, K., Rummery, K. and Keady, J. (2018) 'The lived neighbourhood: Understanding how people with dementia engage with their local environment', *International Psychogeriatrics*, 30(6): 867–80.

Watchman, K. (2017) *Intellectual Disabilities and Dementia: A Guide for Families*, London: Jessica Kingsley.

Westwood, S. and Price, E. (2016) *Lesbian, Gay, Bisexual and Trans* Individuals Living with Dementia: Concepts, Practice and Rights*, Oxford: Routledge.

World Health Organization (2018) *Towards a Dementia Plan: A WHO Guide*, Geneva: WHO.

Index

everyday technologies 24
exclusionary norms 108
exposed, feeling 53–4

F

Facebook 138
facilitated friendships 78–80
familiar, holding on to the 102–4
familiar activities in familiar settings 57
familiar strangers 27, 28
familiarity in places 34–5, 57, 102–3,
   116, 119, 122
family relationships 72–8
fatigue 54, 62
favours, from neighbours 27–32, 39
fear of going outside 116, 128
filmed tours (research methods) 27
fleeting interactions 33–4
   see also gestures of recognition
'fog' 100, 102
Framework of Interplay of Belonging
   and Agency, Aging Well, and the
   Environment 114, 122–30
friendships, maintaining 72–80
Frost, D. 189
fun, having 196

G

Gaber, S.N. 48
Garland-Thomson, R. 108
Genoe, R.M. 195, 196
Geographic Information Systems
   (GIS) 160–85
geographical theory 51
geography 25
gestures of recognition 31, 33, 90, 91,
   92, 118
getting lost 3, 34–5, 58, 92–3,
   99–100, 197
   see also wayfinding
glass walls and doors 55
Global South 210–11
going missing 3, 138
good neighbourly acts 28–9
Goodley, D. 212
GPS trackers 37, 103, 116, 126, 162
Granovetter, M.S. 76
grass roots development 140–59
green spaces 24, 100–1, 108

H

Hägerstrand, T. 161
Handler, S. 213
health care systems 141–2
help, asking for 58–9, 116, 117, 126
heritage sector guidance 201–2
Historic Royal Palaces 201

holidays 191–207
home care services 76, 79, 80, 83
home environment 44–7, 55–6, 69
home tours 70, 98
house moves 44–7
Hulko, W. 212
human rights 5
humour, use of 105–6
hyperstimulation 116

I

identity 114, 115, 117, 120–30,
   196, 212
imagination 101
inclusion in research 152, 189, 211,
   213–14
independence, maintaining 35, 101,
   109–10, 120
Indigenous culture 144, 150, 212
informal interactions 31, 39, 78, 90, 92
informal mentoring 100
Innes, A. 199, 201, 211
insecurity, feelings of 81
Integrative Conceptual Framework
   of Person- Environment
   Exchange 114, 122–30
interdependence 36–7
interdisciplinary dementia
   research 160–85, 214
intergenerational relations 101
intersectionality 212

J

Jeon, Y.-H. 97
'Join Dementia Research' project 189

K

kaleidoscope metaphor 62
Keady, J. 23–4, 211
Klug, K. 201, 203

L

Lamont, R. 195
landmarks 56, 116, 117, 119, 126
languages 144, 150
layouts, logical 55–6
Lefebvre, H. 204, 209
leisure 25, 128, 172–3, 191–207
Lewis, F.M. 48, 146
LGBTQ+ 135–9, 212
Life Changes Trust 95
lifeworld, constriction of 95
Lin, S.Y. 48, 146
living well with dementia 195–7
local history 101–2
local tailored interventions 146, 153–4
localness 35, 37, 38

www.ingramcontent.com/pod-product-compliance
Lightning Source LLC
Chambersburg PA
CBHW070922030426
42336CB00014BA/2505